Beauty is Therapy:

*Memories of the
Traverse City State Hospital*

To Don and Brenda-
Shanks for joining us.
Hope you enjoy the
book-

Earle Steele

Kersten MHains
02-18-01

Beauty is Therapy:

*Memories of the
Traverse City State Hospital*

by Earle E. Steele

as told to Kristen Hains

Denali and Co.
Traverse City

Beauty is Therapy: Memories of the Traverse City State Hospital

ISBN 0-9704778-0-5

LCCN 00-109139

Cover photo courtesy of the Grand Traverse Pioneer and Historical Society.

Foreword

Grandpa once described this venture as "you as granddaughter at my knee, this is rockin' chair format...a sort of Norman Rockwell picture."

Of course, this telling of life and times transpired many times when the rocking chair was in Traverse City and the granddaughter sat listening some 900 miles away in New Jersey.

This project started back in January 1989. I had always delighted in the stories that Grandpa could tell. It suddenly became apparent to me that these were not just stories, they were history. And as Grandpa often said, as the oldest living employee of the Traverse City Regional Psychiatric Hospital, he has many memories of the hospital that at this point are only that.

We boldly started, not knowing where this would lead. From college, I wrote letters and asked questions. He would write back with answers that would trigger new questions. I watched with amazement as history unfolded through the eyes of my grandfather.

I realized that for him, the institution wasn't just a job, but a part of his life. There are few trees on the hospital grounds that were not planted by my grandfather or my great grandfather. Suddenly, this institution, though now closed, became a part of my life. I realized that his memories and recordings of history, coupled with my writing background, could give to others a piece of this area's history.

We could cause an awareness of what the hospital was really like and perhaps erase some of the stereotypes that exist because of present day books and movies.

It is my sincerest wish to keep as much of this in my grandfather's own words. I think the real charm of this book is that it still gives the feeling of grandfather in rocking chair, with granddaughter at his knee.

-Kristen M. Hains

Introduction

The year was March 1922. As nine-year-old Earle Steele left the familiar surroundings of Grand Rapids, he knew very little of a place called Traverse City, only that it would be home, the place his father would accept much-needed employment. Although the Traverse City Regional Psychiatric Hospital had been in existence for nearly 40 years, it was only beginning to come into its own.

Earle Steele traveled by train to Traverse City with his mother, Mamie, to join his father, Edgar H. Steele, who had come to Traverse City in January 1922 to accept the position of Gardener/Florist at the hospital. The move would change Earle's life. A short ten years later, Earle found himself stepping into his father's position. That twist of fate would turn itself into a career that would span some 49 years beyond that.

Beyond what was initially an employment opportunity, Earle Steele would become a part of the history of Traverse City. He would see the institution come full circle, from a thriving institution with a census of 3000 patients in 1943 to a self-sufficient farming operation. He watched as the institution grew, expanded, and eventually, in 1989, closed down.

As much of the grounds now sit unused, awaiting their fate, we must not lose what sits behind closed doors. There is more than dust and chipping paint locked in these buildings. A wealth of history sits untold. If the buildings and grounds could talk, we would all benefit from the knowledge of a time that is a mystery to most of us.

While buildings and grounds can't talk, Earle Steele can tell their stories.

The trees on the grounds of the former Traverse City Regional Psychiatric Hospital, now tall and majestic, were planted by my great grandfather, Edgar Steele in 1928 and, my grandfather, Earle Steele in 1938. They now stand as a symbol of the institution's roots in Traverse City. And although the old buildings and neglected grounds give way to a need for other uses for land and buildings, history should not be lost.

Beauty is Therapy: Memories of the Traverse City State Hospital tells Earle Steele's version of the history of the Traverse City Regional Psychiatric Hospital, as he watched it unfold, first as a child living with his parents on the grounds, then as an employee, and then finally in his retirement as curator of the hospital's museum. His affiliation with the hospital spanned some 66 years. His connection with the hospital passed through the administration of every one of the hospital's Superintendents.

Through letters to me, the story of the hospital began to unfold. Sometimes accompanied by his own illustrations, Grandpa's letters soon began to weave together the history of the hospital.

This book is the compilation of those letters, so that history will not be forgotten.

Beauty is Therapy:

Memories of the
Traverse City State Hospital

Arrival

Little did I know, as I came into Traverse City by train on that cold, blustery March night in 1922, that my direct association with the Traverse City State Hospital would last some sixty years; fifty of those as an employee.

As to the evening of my arrival, Traverse City was just emerging from a three-day blizzard which had added a foot of snow to an accumulation that totaled some four feet. In relation to present wintertime scenes, I find it difficult to give an accurate, true picture of winter times in those early years. No one of this present generation has the knowledge of snow depths or blizzard conditions such as those that existed in the 1920s and 1930s.

To, perhaps, give you a more recent example of life and snow depth and its severity in 1923, I recall a similar storm in January 1978. That particular month produced something akin to that of the old days. If you remember, that was a four-day storm of blowing snow and accumulation that totaled some thirty inches. It provided the first time in some forty six years that I was unable to get to work by dictation of weather conditions.

Back then, snow depths piled up to amounts that towered well above my head (given my normal nine-year-old height), and transportation was strictly of the horse drawn method. To come or go any distance was only accomplished by train and that, at times, was fraught with delays.

Removal of any accumulation was minimal and usually in manual labor efforts… "shovel by hand" a more appropriate title. In the hospital area, most likely due to fear of tragedy from possible fires, snow was removed more avidly there than in the downtown areas. This was accomplished by large working parties of male patients using shovels called "coal scoops." Groups of thirty to forty men would clear walkways, roads, and critical building areas, pile it onto horse-drawn sleighs and take it to field areas for unloading. This took time, of course, but time was what the hospital had in those days. And such work was deemed "therapeutic."

Having spent the prior nine years of my life in southern Michigan, I had never encountered that amount of snow. This probably seems strange to the present generation, but in Traverse City, in earlier years, the bare ground of Spring did not appear until mid-May.

So there was my mother, Mamie, and I getting off the train at the Traverse City depot, located on Union Street, just off of the Sixth Street intersection. We arrived at 11:00 p.m. and were met by my father, Edgar, who had hired the only local taxi that operated in the winter, a 1921 Model T Ford Sedan.

I recall that the immense amount of snow encountered at this time of year was met with dismay on the part of my mother and eager enthusiasm on mine. As I have previously alluded, snow removal in those days was not of today's quality. In fact it was the intention to leave a sufficient quantity on street areas to aid team-drawn sleighs to navigate them. This meant leaving a depth of four or five inches of soft snow on the road. The snow from the previous day having not been removed, the taxi was more than somewhat hindered by the eight to ten inch accumulation. As we floundered from depot to street in unshoveled snow, I suspect my mother looked back to the train, which was then in the process of returning to Grand Rapids, with the desire to be upon it.

I still vividly recall the taxi ride to the hospital grounds and the administration building entrance. The taxi driver was of a burly build. The Fords of those days were of high structure and had high wood-spoked wheels, so as we proceeded up the street, the car was prone to take its own course in the snow. This left the driver madly wrenching the steering wheel to narrowly escape plunging into the roadside's high snow banks. We finally arrived at the administration building's main entrance. The taxi man wouldn't attempt to take us to its doorstep, which meant a final walking distance of some four blocks, again in knee deep snow, before finally arriving at what was to be my home for the next ten years. Even with the hour now very late, I found it hard to get to sleep.

My father had arrived in Traverse City on January 1, 1922, having lost his job in Ann Arbor in the fall of 1921. It proved to be a bad time to be out of work. Seeking employment in the vegetative/floral field during the fall was not easy. It was unusual that my father lost his job, as he was well-known state wide for his skill in commercial chrysanthemum and rose growing methods. Apparently, it was because the greenhouse complex in Ann Arbor was a corporation owned enterprise with a local lawyer in charge. His only knowledge of greenhouse work was the money he expected to come in on a weekly basis. My father faithfully helped with the profit and had upgraded the floral sales greatly in the two years he had worked there as supervisor.

At some point the lawyer was contacted by a florist who claimed that he could outdo my father's ability by 100 percent in one year. My father was let go the next day, and began earnestly seeking a new cultural style that would tie in with what he was known for state-wide, which brought him to Traverse City to assume the position of Florist-Gardener Supervisor in charge of greenhouses and garden areas. My mother and I arrived later in order to accommodate a renovation program of the cottage assigned to the florist. The renovation lasted from January 1 until March 15, 1922 and included new heating and interior decorating. The house, still in existence although unused at present, was built, I believe, in 1890. The gardener at that time was a man of Swiss nationality and he had a growing family. A humorous story told, with some doubt to its truth, was that, as he added a new member to his family, a new room was added to the home. I can vouch for some truth in that story by reason of room arrangement—there were five and only one bathroom. What a crisis that must have presented at times, but it actually did not effect our lives at the time.

Lighting was in the early style with drop cords from ceiling outlets in all rooms and no electrical outlets. You can well imagine that no outlets in the kitchen curtailed any electrical fixtures. The stove was gas, with a wood burning element, which my mother would use when all stove burners were in use. I marvel at the meals my mother created as she totally disregarded any inconvenience. My mother's washing machine was primitive in that it was run by a gasoline motored driving machine. The machine was large and cumbersome and was initially placed in the bathroom which took up critical space for bathing and other urgent bathroom necessities. I can't remember any frustration on her part while living there, but in light of today's conveniences, how did she do it?

We were the first to move in with a car. The humor in that came when the hospital carpentry division built the attached garage unit with no knowledge of how large a car we owned. Subsequently, a base wall and floor of poured concrete had to be removed and redone. We must remember this was still a predominantly "horse and buggy" time. The doors to our home were never locked or barricaded, even considering our close proximity to the patient wards.

But, back to my arrival in Traverse City. The next morning, I was awakened by the hospital's power plant whistle which started the day's activities in maintenance sections. I would be involved with that whistle for some 40 years after that first awakening. Its shrill voice was heard at 7:00 a.m., 11:30 a.m., and 5:00 p.m., when it closed out the day's activities. It was also used in Monday morning fire drill practices. By sounding short bursts of the whistle, it would announce where on the grounds the drill was to be held.

Breakfast was provided in a nearby kitchen, as a courtesy, by hospital authorities who knew of our late arrival and that no foods were in the pantry area. Having explored our new home from top to bottom, I elected to go outside. Floundering delightedly in the deep snow, I suddenly became aware of a group of thirty to fifty men with large scoop shovels clearing a sidewalk nearby. A few, having spotted me, began shouting hello at me. I just stood silently, watching from a distance. This was my first exposure to patient group activity which, indeed, became commonplace through the many years thereafter.

Just then, a team of horses pulling a large sleigh came along the roadbed directly in front of our residence. It gave me my first experience of the friendliness that existed between employees, regardless of department, and patients. The driver of the team stopped the sleigh saying, "Hello, How about riding with me? I shall be coming back this way." I didn't know this man, or the situation, but I was fascinated by the chance to ride on the horse drawn sleigh, something I had never done before. So, without notification of parent, which would be duly corrected later that day, I clambered onto the sleigh and off we went. As I sat by the driver, he asked me the usual questions of name, age and how I liked Traverse City.

Getting onto the sleigh, I had not noticed that there was a series of large, metal cans stashed there, which turned out to be milk cans of fifty gallon size. These were being delivered to several hospital kitchens. This delivery medium, which the driver called 'the cookie wagon,' delivered all the food items to each kitchen area, including meats, milk, and baked goods, a method that was in used until about 1938.

As we progressed from kitchen to kitchen the cooks in these areas spotted me on the sleigh and the very unusualness of someone so young being on board evoked the question, "Who's your new helper?" This produced the explanation as to who I was. I would later return home and rush into the house to relate my adventure to mother, which resulted in a discussion as to the advisability of letting her know my whereabouts at all times, which was agreed to on my part as the right thing to do.

Another memory of riding the 'cookie' wagon was in the late afternoons to deliver milk from the dairy to the kitchens. I'd climb onto the sleigh as it went by and ride around. This involved delivery to four kitchens scattered about the grounds. The furthest kitchen was located in the area now known as Munson Medical Center. This particular team of horses had belonged to Dr. James D. Munson, the hospital superintendent. He had advanced to the automotive age and, therefore, donated his team to the hospital work force. They were not only lightweight, but also high-spirited. Upon getting to the Munson area kitchen, they seemed to know it was the last stop, and when we started the return trip, they proceeded "full tilt," with the driver vainly attempting to slow them down. I would busily dodge empty milk cans to be returned to the dairy as they slid from side to side on the sleigh. As for getting off in front of my house-forget it- it was all the way to the barn, which was approximately one-half mile away. I really didn't mind. In fact, my juvenile mind compared it to a horse race.

In the afternoon, my mother and I ventured down to my father's workstation in the greenhouse, which consisted of five glass houses and a large workroom. This was built in 1892 and was not in the best of shape, so it did challenge my father in productive qualities.

In the following few days, before my mother insisted that it was time to get me back into school, my father insisted that I accompany him in a visit to the administrative office areas to meet, and get acquainted with, personnel to whom he had spoken about me. So, early one morning, office to office we went. Upon arrival in each office area, I met office clerks (mostly women), male bookkeepers, and telephone desk operators. I was made to feel very welcome and many of these people remained friends for years to follow. When my father took me into the office of Dr. Munson, I found him to be a very gracious and gentle person. If he happened to meet me in my sidewalk "wagon traveling," he would always stop and visit. Even in busy times, when he was checking ward areas, he would stop and visit, always interested in what I was doing. I think part of his interest was due to the fact that he had only one son, who was born during the early years of the institution. The son graduated from high school and, it being the years of World War I, had joined the army. He tragically perished during training camp from a flu epidemic in 1917, and this, indeed, was a tragedy for Dr. Munson. I learned in later years, while operating the Traverse City Regional Psychiatric hospital museum that Dr. Munson's son had a "high school buddy" who was often in Dr. Munson's Hospital apartment. This person was later to be known as Dr.

6

Edwin Thirlby, a noted local surgeon and physician. Dr. Thirlby always maintained that Dr. Munson urged him into a medical career at a time when he was not sure of what career he desired. Two days later, much to my chagrin, my mother, who was ever mindful that I'd missed a great amount of school, hastened to get me started again. I'd missed nearly the entire school year in the transition from first Ann Arbor to Grand Rapids, and then Grand Rapids to Traverse City. I had entered the fourth grade in Ann Arbor in the fall of 1921. I was not the greatest of scholars, and all this transition didn't enhance the situation.

I was taken to register at the Union Street school, located where the St. Francis Church is now located. I lasted about a week in the fourth grade and was then returned to the third grade level. This teacher, bless her soul, was so right to move me. Union Street School, at the corner of Union and Thirteenth Streets was later demolished when Glenn Loomis Elementary School replaced it. Upon entering the eighth grade, which was considered junior high, I moved to Eighth Street. The building that housed eighth and ninth graders burned down in 1934, and just my luck, I graduated in 1933! The fire caused an immediate problem as to where to hold classes. Interestingly, a historical society's memoir collection showed some classes were held in the basement of the Sixth Street library, and some, believe it or not, were held in the home of Perry Hannah, now a funeral home. My lifestyle was peculiar in a sense because, as an only child living in a secluded area, I think I "grew up" a lot sooner than normal.

One memory that I recall most vividly is the winter times. In those times, storms often left one "holed up" in a warm house, reading. Bored with that, I would occasionally go down to the greenhouse while my father worked. Being in the greenhouse, in floral areas surrounded by greenery, helped to temporarily take away the weather conditions outside. Perhaps it was this activity that was the beginning association for what ultimately became my own career.

I still recall the clear, still moonlit nights outside. There was one night in the early 1930s, shortly after graduation from high school, when a friend and I went skiing. The temperature read thirty degrees below zero, but it was clear and still. I remember skiing through wooded areas where the deep frost had penetrated the bark on the trees to the point that inside, the bark would freeze, then explode with the sound of a rifle shot. It was startling, to say the least, when that would happen to a tree close to you. Strangely enough, it never seemed to damage the trees.

I remember well every aspect of winter. Beginning in about 1925, people had moved from horse-drawn vehicles to cars. They tried to operate cars year round, which necessitated better snow clearance from street areas. By the same token, some snow had to be left for farmers who came to town via horse and sleigh. So, during early spring thaws, melting roadbeds would promote car tracks some four to six inches deep. These would freeze up again at night. Woe to the early morning motorist as he hit the streets and its many tracks. Inevitably, the front wheels would set in one set of tracks, the rear wheels in another. This would result in a sideways journey down the street. And, if for some reason the car would jump these ruts, they merely changed sideways directions. Getting through an intersection became even more of a challenge, as the criss-cross from all streets presented many challenges in navigation, usually to the detriment of reaching said destination.

In the days of my elementary education, getting to school was achieved through team power and I wondered sometimes, in severe weather, how the horses knew where to go and they always found the way. I suspect that method of "delivery" created some envy among my peers. The teamster in charge had strict orders that no one but hospital employees' children was to ride. I think this was brought on by the fear of possible injury occurring to riders who were not considered 'legal'. I always felt sorry for the driver, as he would have to ride on the rear of the sleigh and be exposed to the wrath of children's snowballs. The children allowed to ride were protected beneath a canvas cover and nestled in a straw laden floor. Occasionally, a misdirected snowball bouncing off a horse would cause an accelerated ride until the teamster could regain control. The farm manager, whose two daughters traveled with me to school, was a former teacher and, consequently, very adamant that we attend school promptly and daily. This led to our going to school in stormy times when we would be the only students there. Kids living but a block away would stay at home, but most of the teachers were single and rented available rooms close by so, they were always there on time.

Wintertime travel was not easy. Grocery supplies were delivered by horse drawn sleigh from small grocery stores in neighborhood areas all across town. I recall seeing enclosed wagons delivering milk to residential routes very early in the morning. A minimum temperature control was maintained by a kerosene lantern set up in the wagon. Milk left on the porches was, hopefully, retrieved immediately, in that milk left out to the elements would be subject to a strange phenomenon- freezing would force the milk to push up on its cardboard cap so that when it was retrieved, it would be in a solid state of protrusion. Sometimes this would raise it one to two inches above the cap area.

The State Hospital had its own railroad track and received many, many cars of coal. It went into service, in 1914 and enabled the hospital to cut shipping costs of materials from outside of the immediate area, such as coal, dry goods, clothing and medical supplies.

My sole interest in the railroad on one of those days, as a nine year old, was to retrieve from the shipping list a large coaster wagon given to me as a Christmas present when we were in Ann Arbor. My anxiety in waiting at the hospital receiving area was only outdone by my frustration from my inability to use it immediately, the result of mass quantities of snow. In dry and good times, that wagon was my constant companion and did accompany me as I "tooled around" the grounds on the many sidewalks.

An interesting side note is that this institution was the first one, of the three existing at that time, with electrical power. This initiated the necessity to establish a power plant with generators driven by steam, and the need to increase the size of the furnace heating plant (Boiler Room). The wiring was two wire type and went through the underground utility tunnel, from building to building, although some wiring was carried above ground to buildings in outer areas. In the beginning, the decision to have electricity was met with much opposition from all officials. Their fear was of potential threat of fire. Fire in institutional buildings was prevalent in tragedies encountered in early hospitals. Our hospital had a roster of four employees who were electricians. In later times the hospital carried some ten employees in this department. The electricity was only used in critical areas and then minimally. The only switching equipment (keys) was carried by ward personnel.

The hospital power plant, which generated its own electrical power as well as providing heat and hot water, would burn sixty five tons of coal in a twenty four hour period in the coldest weather. It had its own waterwells that produced, at maximum, six hundred thousand gallons in twenty four hours. The wells are still in existence, but have been capped off. I can still see car after car of coal being pushed up to be unloaded adjacent to the power plant. Coal was on order year round. Summer accumulation, when the need was less, would find it stacked up some three stories high.

Coal was the major heating source. It was, in fact, the only method in early times, in that oil was primarily in kerosene mode, and was used mainly for cooking. Coal was in a large lump form brought to town via boat. It was dispensed to households from dockside coal yards. The area now known as Open Space was a former coal and lumberyard known as the Hannah Lay Company yard. As the supply diminished in that area, coal was then brought in by rail and dispensed from a storage yard in the railroad area. This was in the vicinity of where the Cone Drive Gear plant is now located, just off from Cass Street.

Winters were always enjoyable even though entertainment was sparse. Radio was in its infancy and television was unheard of. In many cases, travel modes were limited as many stored their automobiles for the winter. If this was the case, your choices were walk, or take a taxi. My father, an avid movie fan, would, once a month, requisition a taxi, and off we would go to attend the local movie theater, which carried the odd name of Dreamland. It was located about where, at present, is the U an I Lounge on Front Street. Admission cost was ten cents, and for an adult, it was twenty five cents. My father was partial to Westerns and we became fans of William S. Hart, Tom Mix and Hoot Gison, the cowboys stars of those times.

I remember coming home from the theater via taxi one cold, clear, February night. Coming up Union Street and passing over the bridge, we saw many people standing on the walks. Many flashing lights were followed by the fire department, who were desperately trying to put out huge fire that ultimately consumed Hannah Lay gristmill. The huge clouds of smoke and steam rose high in the air above the building. Union Street was aglow with lights that marked the path of fire trucks lining the curbside. Due to snow accumulation, they couldn't get close to the building.

Another source of entertainment was the hospital library. While small in size, its contents were donated varieties and provided a Mecca of reading. This instilled within me a great enthusiasm for reading. As the weather cleared up and automotive travel could be had, there was also the library on Sixth Street.

By way of commerce, Traverse City was geared primarily toward the cherry industry in summer, and then in winter, it was pretty much "roll up the sidewalks." After this, one just waited for spring. Of work sources, the Iron Works was the largest and the State Hospital was the largest employer. Neither ever lacked of a needy field of employment seekers, due to the fact that many farmers and hired hands experienced loss of work in winter and would hire on as an attendant nurse. This was done with the understanding that it would only be from November until April. This was agreeable to hospital officials and was the mode of hired help until civil service in 1938. At that point, hiring tactics took a different turn.

Of personal recreational involvement, radio was just coming into popularity. It was not in existence for us, but I remember friends of my parents having a large console type radio. On Sunday evenings, we would often be invited to listen to Eddie Cantor and Ed Wynn, as well as the news, and were fascinated by this new concept.

The difficulty was in the fact that good radio reception demanded some pretty extensive antenna equipment. Eventually my father agreed to have a radio, but just a small table model. Our proximity to the hospital power plant would totally ruin reception at times due to electrically made static, generally at the time of the special program that I desired to hear. That radio was a great source of enjoyment for my mother, who spent a great amount of time at home while Dad was at work and I was at school.

I continued to use the public library as an amusement source. In addition to this, my friend, Walt, and I would enjoy skiing and tobogganing in wintertime and tennis, hiking, and swimming in the summer.

With year-round ability to get around, thanks to our automobile, my father was insistent that movie attendance downtown be accomplished by way of the offerings at the Lyric Theater, which was consumed by fire in 1944. In those days, the films changed often-every day of the week-and, amazingly, there was live vaudeville on Thursday and Friday nights. We attended every one. Sometimes, if the film playing was one which my father appreciated greatly, we would attend the second night's showing as well. This was more likely to happen during the winter months, and early friendship with the theater manager provided occasional free access which, no doubt, had some bearing as well.

In summertime, the family would get into the car and proceed downtown, the first stop being Wahl's candy and ice cream store on Union Street. Three ice cream cones were purchased, then it was on to the railroad station just south of Eighth at Franklin Street, to watch the resort special on its way south from Petoskey. You would have to see it to appreciate the scene. A big steam locomotive, followed by several cars and some Pullman coaches carried resorters on their way back to Chicago, many just retiring for what would be an overnight trip for them.

Another amusement source would be to go down to the boat dock which was situated where Clinch Marina is now located. In the 1920s and 1930s, larger passenger boats would dock there at least three times a week. They came out of Chicago, with frequent stops all the way up the

West Michigan coastline. It was another method for tourists to get to northern Michigan vacation sites. Mackinac Island was the furthest point of travel. Again it was interesting to watch the people get off, make a hurried trip up town, and then hurry back to the ship as it would only make a two-hour stop. The ships stayed only long enough to load and unload freight. In season, sweet and sour cherries were on their way to the Chicago market as this method provided a fast route. With highways of minimal quality and quantity, most freight was handled by mode of boat or train.

During times of inclement weather, I spent a great deal of time in the greenhouses. There were five patients (also called residents) who worked year round. These residents were men who came from either farming or carpentry backgrounds. Most visitors and much of the outside public would wonder why residents often seemed so content. I think this was due, in part, to their age and the fact that they were quite satisfied to let someone else do the caring. As the elderly passed on, I saw a younger, more belligerent, generation enter the hospital.

As time went on, I spent more and more time in the greenhouses. Regretfully, I didn't pay too much attention to that which would have been of great benefit to me in the coming years. If only I had known this would become my lifetime employment, I might have taken a few notes along the way.

My routine was basically "straight to school and straight home," which gave me little opportunity to make friends. I did meet two boys who became close friends. One still is, the other perished in a plane accident. I manufactured my own entertainment sources, which consisted of stream fishing on hospital grounds and hiking tours. There's not much of the grounds or areas of land adjacent that I don't know thoroughly, even yet.

I didn't necessarily mind that I didn't have a great number of friends my own age on the grounds. It wasn't until Junior High that I began to entertain thoughts of wondering what my classmates did after school. I often wonder what might have happened if I had been more outward and attended more functions. My mother tried to get me to participate in band, but I defeated that endeavor. I showed more interest in illustration and drawing, and the art teacher urged me to participate and enter schooling to enhance my capabilities. I thought, as I got further into high school, that I might pursue a career in commercial art. However, I had a friend who was a commercial artist who encouraged me to seek other employment.

In my later teen years, during summertime, I would work within the greenhouse or garden area, more for something to do. My interest was not in pursuance of agricultural elements. Looking back, if I had any particular element that I thought of pursuing it was to be a National Park Ranger or some area related to forestry.

For me, 1923 and 1924 flew by. For the most part, I was healthy, with the exception of when I was thirteen and underwent surgery for appendicitis. The appendicitis was initially misdiagnosed, which ultimately led to an exploratory surgery which produced the "villainous" appendix. It was such a severe surgical procedure that I was out of school and confined to my bed for four months. You can well imagine the frustration that confinement produced in a thirteen-year-old. At the time of my surgery, the hospital did have a fair-sized library. A resident of the State Hospital maintained the library. He was an elderly gentleman who was asked by the superintendent to supply me with books that might be interesting to a thirteen-year-old. The poor man had a minimal youthful selection as most of books were donated. He did the best he could, and didn't deliver just one book, but twenty to thirty at a time. I was hospitalized from December 1 until December 24. I was brought home by ambulance and required to stay in bed until March 1. This time, I kept my schoolwork up through 'homework.' I did have problems the rest of the elementary years as I was not a good student. In 1927 I started wearing glasses, in order to correct nearsightedness.

In the fall of 1929, I moved on to Central School. While this did bring about different school classmates, the peer group was about the same caliber. The fact that I still resided in the realm and center of the

Hospital meant I was a loner. In afterthought, maybe I should have exhibited a more outgoing demeanor, but that just wasn't my nature.

As I approached high school graduation, I suddenly began to realize that I'd not bettered myself in preparation for college. It had been my parent's hope that I would attend the University of Michigan. My brother lived in Ann Arbor and had volunteered to help me with the room and board, which meant I would be responsible for the tuition. By neglecting my schoolwork and not attempting to find summer employment, I had two strikes against me, so that took care of college. But, all things being equal, I couldn't have gone anyway with the economy still so desperate. As a family, we were very fortunate that we had furnished living quarters and utilities, and most foods. As the Depression dragged on, other family members, living in the Detroit area, came upon difficult times with no jobs and no unemployment insurance. My folks felt a duty to help. With so many families out of work locally, the suggestion was made for me to stay at home in hopes that the economy would rebound and better times would return. So home I stayed.

The Hospital: 1923-1934

At the time, Traverse City might have been better registered as a village, as opposed to a town. It had a Post Office, which gave it priority as a city. In productive areas, it had an Iron Works which made heavy metal objects such as fire hydrants and manhole covers, as well as a vegetable and fruit packaging factory. These were the only year round industries of the town. There were several wood manufacturing companies that were thriving until the lumber sources of the area succumbed to loss by harvest, when they either expired on the spot or moved to other areas where material was still available. There was also an automobile factory, which did a good business for awhile and then went bankrupt, as did many fledgling enterprises in auto manufacturing in the late teens and early 1920s. There are several historical accountings, now in print, which detail these companies and their effects on Traverse City development.

Of some 6,000 people who were residents of Traverse City, there were an additional 2200 people who were patients at the State Hospital. While their upkeep was supplied through hospital purchases from city sources, they were not included in census counts. Possibly the reasoning was that they were not actually citizens of Traverse City, having come from other counties.

The possibility of jobs and revenue may be the reason why there was a mental institution this far north in Michigan. So back we go to the late 1880s, 1881 to be exact. An early settler, named Perry Hannah, became a lumber baron and consequently the area's first millionaire. He was also known as "the father of Traverse City," because he was interested in seeing Traverse City become a large and forceful element in the growth of northern Michigan.

As the lumbering industry began to fold due to the exhaustion of pinewood, he could foresee that Traverse City might fade out just as other communities had. In 1881, Mr. Hannah was a member of the State Legislative body. The state was contemplating adding another mental facility to the two already in existence in southern Michigan, the only two within the state.

Kalamazoo's institution was established in 1870 and the one in Pontiac followed in 1878. Distance played a factor for those in need of hospitalization and so the thinking in legislative circles was to establish the next mental hospital somewhere in the northern tier of the state. The need was great, and the thought was to build another hospital in central northern Michigan. There being no such unit in this area, the mentally ill were cared for within the home or, if violent in nature, the county jail.

Kalamazoo and Pontiac serviced only the southern portion of the state. As mental illness was not afflicting only that part of the state, patients from the northern tier were transported to these southern institutions. Travel modes were very primitive at the time and because the existing institutions were very overcrowded, the need to locate another facility in another area became even more apparent. A three member group of legislators was formed to assess where would be the most convenient location for all concerned. Hannah, at that time the representative from Grand Traverse county and areas in the northern Lower Peninsula, was made chairman of this group. When his attendance was required at meetings held in Lansing, he would walk, the best travel means to get to areas in southern Michigan. He would take with him an Indian guide and it would take three weeks to get there.

Some 15 locations were originally considered and this group was narrowed to five- Greenville, Manistee, Big Rapids, Reed City and Traverse City. Traverse City was the final selection in that the ground type was excellent for heavy building construction, plus it provided a large plot of land at a cheap price. It also offered a sufficient source of water. Many residents of Traverse City realized the potential value of the hospital being located in Traverse City. They knew it would not only provide employment, but also generate purchases in the mercantile area. Many citizens contributed monetarily to a fund to purchase the necessary land, and Perry Hannah donated a great deal of his own land.

The honorable Mr. Hannah, being aware of current problems through his legislative association, sought to assure the hospital's location in Traverse City. The hospital began with a $400,000 appropriation from the state legislator. After much deliberation and final funding being approved, construction began in 1883. On November 5, 1885, the first patient entered the new hospital, and that term remained in effect until 1978 when the mentally ill were called "residents." (This was deemed a more respectful title). The hospital was originally named "Northern Michigan Asylum for the Insane in Traverse City Michigan," a title that was maintained until the year of 1911 when it gave way to Traverse City State Hospital. My understanding of the name change was that it was the result of a need in the business and records department to expedite bookkeeping.

The hospital was essentially built in the heavily forested northern Michigan wilderness, and this meant an immediate need for a water source and land clearance for the building of barn areas, grazing land and garden areas. The institution opened for business in November of that year, serving some 39 counties then in existence from Bay City across to Muskegon and then north to Mackinaw City.

Interestingly enough, the first building, along with several others, is still in existence. It was thought that this unit, which was constructed to house some 550 people, would last indefinitely into the future. But the superintendent, Dr. Munson found himself back in two years pleading with the legislature to construct more housing units to alleviate overcrowding. So as the years advanced, more cottage units were added and with that, accordingly, additional maintenance workers.

That first building was built on a small clearing that had to be enlarged to accommodate the total building and ultimately the succeeding individual cottages. The land clearance was achieved by patient labor force, a therapeutic program strongly advocated by Dr. Munson.

Shortly after the original Building 50 was completed, many more patients from southern Michigan arrived. Dr. Munson immediately saw the need for additional space and sought legislative aid to increase the size of Building 50. While this took much persuasion, Dr. Munson finally gained the necessary help to add two wings, one on each side of the building. The appropriations for Building 50 was $450,000.00.

Additional land was cleared for agricultural purposes. It was necessary to first acquire pastureland for the growing dairy head, and then to procure land for vegetable cropping. This use of the land was a necessity because money appropriations to operate the institution from state legislation were very meager and primarily went for utility costs, such as coal, medical supplies and employee wages. It became mandatory that food supplies be augmented by what could be grown and stored for use. The hospital also maintained root cellar storage facilities and mush canning processes.

The first land clearance did not bring forth a great quantity of fruits and vegetables. The need was to be self-supportive and as soon as possible. Dr. Munson desired not only food sources, but lawn and shrubbery placement. Though it wasn't until 1902 that appropriations were made and garnered to build a greenhouse.

Land was continually purchased and developed agriculturally as the institution grew in size and consequent needs. In the early 1950s, the total land comprised some 1600 acres-of which 65 acres were lawn campus areas. As the institution grew, its cost in maintenance likewise increased. The cost of construction left little money for operating costs which meant the hospital needed to be more and more self-sufficient. This was primarily accomplished in food supply, which turned to dairy head and truck garden, plus orchard area development. Dr. Munson, had been a farm boy in youth and felt that farming could be of great benefit, therapeutically speaking, giving the mentally ill something to do which might take their minds off their problems.

One must remember that in early days of the hospital it took much courage, determination and skill to acquire the necessities. My father's hiring, I believe, was by reason of the dire need for the most expert supervisory personnel. The hospital needed to be as self-sufficient as possible and this had to be accomplished in a manner that offset the insufficient appropriations allotted to run the institution.

This is how the Steele family ultimately became residents of Northern Michigan. My father's job title was listed as gardener/florist. The gardener portion detailed the field crop area including vegetables and small fruits. The florist pertained to the greenhouse floral area including potted plants utilized in indoor decor, ferns, large leafed greenery, cut flowers (carnations and roses) and the growing of bedding plants for the planting of the many flower beds on the grounds in summer. Prior to our coming to Traverse City, the hospital officials had experienced difficulty in finding a suitable head gardener and florist to take charge of that department. Dr. Munson, unable to find suitable local "talent," contacted a bank president friend in Grand Rapids, hoping to find a suitable candidate. It so happened that this bank president was a former schoolmate of my father. My father, being out of work at the time, encountered his banker friend to ask if he knew of any job possibilities. You can probably surmise the outcome.

Beauty is Therapy

As I mentioned before the lack of state financial appropriations forced the hospital to become self supportive and immediately had to begin the farming process. Dairy needs were addressed first, and then, as fast as land could be cleared, vegetable and fruit crops had to be installed. This required a greenhouse to start vegetable plants, thus the need for a Head Gardener.

This program tied in directly with an early theory of Dr. Munson. He had a life long theory which, in essence, could be titled "Beauty is Therapy." Most people not connected to the Institution couldn't understand it because the general public assumed that mental institutions were more like a prisons. Dr. Munson held to his theory, believing that work was an excellent therapeutic program. Patients were involved from day one in land clearing, not only for field areas and grounds proper, but also for ongoing building construction. They contributed greatly to the labor force, though building construction was of contract basis and no patient labor was involved. Some construction, which was handled by the hospital itself, did involve the use of patient labor, but they were never "paid" for this labor as it was deemed part of their therapy. In later years, this became an issue and eventually the patient labor groups were discontinued.

Patient labor was necessary as the institution was growing. Downtown citizens who often witnessed patients in fieldwork assumed that it was forced. This patient workforce provided me with my first exposure to labor party grouping. In all the years of witnessing groups or even being in charge of one, I never heard one complaint of having to work- to all, it was an opportunity to get off the ward areas. Those who chose not to work, were then placed on a non-working class ward, and if physical disabilities were an issue, those individuals were free from work.

The Hospital was constructed out of a wooded wilderness. Everything adjacent to the Hospital buildings was surrounded by raw land — stumps, stones and rough soil. Dr. Munson's plan for beautifying the grounds adjacent to the newly constructed buildings began in 1888 and continued for many years.

First came stump removal and grading of lawn areas, then after land clearance, the planting trees and shrubbery adjacent to buildings and driveways. An ornamental pool was placed on the grounds and lawn benches and chairs were added, was the beginning of Dr. Munson's Arboretum, starting in the mid 1890's.

The Doctor often visited distant States and would bring back several young trees to add to his arboretum. He continued to do so until a few years before his retirement in 1924. Many of his selected trees are still living, but some have died due to age or lack of care.

Over the years, I have taken many groups of interested school children and their teachers, Boy Scouts and other groups on lecture tours of the Aboretum, often to identifiy leafs in the fall.

In the mid sixties, Dr. Duane Sommerness, the hospital superintendent at the time, ordered metal name tags be put on all trees on the campus area. A Horticultural Professor, from Michigan State University, was brought in to properly identify each tree. Dr. Sommerness, through his Publicity Agent, Ohmer Curtis, made known to the local newspaper that the trees were so named and the public was welcome to come see and enjoy them. This became a boon to the local high school teachers, who would make it a field trip for students to collect leaves, twigs and seed formations.

Some of the unusual varieties of trees that Dr. Munson brought back from his many business trips were English Hawthorne, which had a very pretty bloom in early summer. Along with this group was the Ginkgo tree. There are four total. These trees were not totally hardy, but still would survive our severe winters. I once saw a group of Ginkgo trees on the White House grounds in Washington D.C.. I could not believe their gigantic size. Ninety feet in height and a four-five foot trunk diameter. Our trees were not so majestic. One could put their arms around them and they were not more than twenty feet high.

My father did an immense amount of planting in this area during his years of employment. Later years, between the 1940's and 1980's and prior to my retirement, I did much maintenance to keep these trees healthy.

I have been very humbled by the tree that was planted in my honor for my 50 years of service on the grounds. This happened during the fall of 1998. The fact that my tree was placed near the Arboretum area and on the grounds owned by the Pavilions and Grand Traverse County leads me to believe that the Arboretum will be further developed on the Pavilions grounds. There were some trees removed to make room for the new Pavilions building, but for each one, another tree of like variety was promised to be planted.

Consequent with the rapid growth of the census of the patients was the increased necessity for more food production, such as the institutional farming was doing. Food production was necessary not only in quantity, but quality as well. Small and large fruit production was vital to hospital welfare as the hospital was totally dependent on agriculture. This was due to the fact that legislative appropriations were very meager and allocated to medical salaries and clothing needs.

More land was cleared for field crop production, which necessitated the need for more labor, both residential and employee. It was vital that competent supervisory personnel be acquired. In the beginning years, the local employees were well versed in farm production, and as the institution grew in size, so did the need for more educated personnel.

While most land clearance was accomplished through patient work force, I remember being 12 years old in 1927 and watching a man setting dynamite explosives under stumps in an area along Division St and on the Eleventh street section leading into the grounds. I was on my home from school, and curiosity compelled me to stop and watch. I saw a man touch off a fuse, madly race away some distance and then "BOOM!"— up went the stump in the air well above the ground. All that was left was a splintered stump to be hauled away, and large holes from the dynamite charges. This also left "pick n' shovel" repair by resident crew members supervised by attendant ground supervisor. I was told "get lost" by the "dynamiter" unless I treasured having a stump or parts there of land on my head. I promptly left the area.

The institution had a large farm, well away from the main area. It included cherries, apples, plums and pears. The original land purchased was utilized in crop production of animal feed such as hay and oats, as a well as food for the herd of some 400 Holstein cattle. If there is question as to why some fruits were grown in great quantity, it was simply because there was quite a bit of processing involved. The hospital maintained a large canning kitchen for fruit processing. Sour cherries were mainly canned in great quantity for pie making. During the off season, apples were used for applebutter and applesauce and canned for pies. In the area of vegetables, tomatoes yielded some four thousand bushels, and were canned as catsup and tomato juice. Many tons of cabbage were produced, resulting in some sixty five barrels of sauerkraut. This balance provided weekly kitchen supplies for stew, coleslaw and boiled dinners. Beets, carrots, onions, celery, rutabaga and squash were kept on hand in great quantity.

The time period of 1926 to 1929 demonstrated the transition from the "horse and buggy" era to the early mechanization in all areas. More and more people were purchasing cars, and trucks quickly became the mode of freight travel. Buses were somewhat primitive in style compared to today's Greyhounds. City officials were required to be more diligent in winter snow removal as cars were in use year round. By this time mechanization, had taken hold in various hospital areas as passenger cars, assisting in patient transfer from building to building. Prior to this, when it was necessary to transfer a patient to another institution, any travel to a distant institution was accomplished via the railroad. You can also suspect the problem if the person in transfer was uncooperative. In this instance, it required two employee personnel to assist in delivery, so the advent of automobile as a method of transportation did much to curtail cost factors.

The farm still maintained the horse-drawn methods in farming activities, as well as in food delivery and garbage pick-up. The farm manager was very adamant in scorning the use of tractors in the fields. In fact, when a business official demanded that he try one, he promptly sought the wettest spot in the field, and told the driver to "Bury it!" which the driver did very effectively. This led to no mechanization, agriculturally speaking, until 1936.

You may wonder what the institution was like at this time. The need was ever growing, and a census count of 2200 patients in 1924 had risen to 2700 and a subsequent waiting list was developing. While medical personnel had increased, treatment programs were primarily psychoanalytical which bred to the treatment that ultimately destroyed the institutional form of housing and caring. This method ultimately got the title of "warehousing" of the mentally ill, which, in essence, was true, but it served to assist those who are now known as "street people."

Any institution that houses so many mentally ill residents must be closely regimented. All activities, including sleeping, eating, work habits, recreation and entertainment required guidance. Consequently, the caregivers became regimented and the nursing staff and maintenance suppliers were housed along with residents.

Our cottage was situated some 50-100 yards away from the nearest cottage building, which housed anywhere from 80-100 male residents who worked in various areas around the hospital grounds, generally in maintenance areas. Some residents had grounds privileges that allowed them to get to job stations while others were more "guarded" and worked mostly in group labor areas. This consisted of some 30-50 residents working in group assignment who were watched and guided.

These groups were fed in a central dining hall. Meal times were 6:30 a.m., 12:00 p.m. and 5:30 p.m. Patient activities included church, which was a mandatory function for all that were able, and was held on Sunday as well as holidays. Monday nights were movie nights, and once a month on Friday night, a dancing/social was held which would mark the only contact between male and female residents.

It had long been the desire of Dr. Munson to properly house and care for tubercular afflicted patients in separate a building. In the past, they had always been placed among the other patients who were not afflicted. Munson tried for several years prior to his retirement in June 1924 to gain appropriations in order to establish separate units. Dealing with the state legislature of those times went without success until 1931-1932 when appropriations were rendered and two buildings constructed. One was built for tubercular housing, the other was called a bed-patient cottage, specifically for general physical ailments and the terminally ill. These two buildings are still in existence. An interesting note is that these two units could, and did, care for some 300 patients in the beginning years and were functional up until 1982. It would be 1939 before the next large unit was built.

Some of the hospital buildings were constructed in the early days of my youth. The grounds existed from Sixth Street, west of Elmwood Avenue to approximately where the present Meijers store is today. Silver Lake Road bisected the field areas on the southern section, and the barns were built near Silver Lake Road. The cottage buildings were clustered near Building 50. The building areas made up 65 acres of the grounds. The field area which included the dairy herd and planted crops covered some 1600 acres. In the 1950s, the State Mental Health Department decided not to pay patients for their labor and therefore discontinued the patient work force. This decision meant much of the land was sold off. The land directly adjacent to the buildings was sold to Munson Hospital and to Grand Traverse County.

In 1925, Dr. Munson won his long cherished dream of a general public hospital, which in later years was named after him. The building was still a part of the State Hospital property and was state owned. In 1947, Munson Hospital was turned over to a corporate group and the state relinquished their property ownership. I vividly remember the days of construction. It was a two-story building, lengthy in structure, and the labor source was State Hospital patients. The state hired engineers and architects. Other than that, State Hospital maintenance employees and building materials were supplied by the State Hospital.

The next structure built was the Women's Dining Room building. This was situated next to the cottage that housed the female patients. The second floor of this building housed an auditorium and was jointly used for Chapel services. This building was built in 1927 and demolished in 1994. The Men's Dining Room was constructed and opened for use in 1916. This unit serviced all the male cottages to the south side. The dining room was built and nestled neatly between Cottages twenty four and twenty six. Prior to the communal dining rooms being built, kitchen and dining areas were housed in the individual cottages.

To the south, was cottage 28 which was the men's geriatric ward. To the southwest of cottage 28, some 100 feet away, was cottage 30, which was designated as a workers' cottage. The men in this cottage assisted in field work in season and snow removal in winter time. This cottage housed some 60-90 men, the higher count being in 1943 when the Hospital was extremely overcrowded. The next cottage to come along, some 60 feet beyond Cottage 32 was the men's tuberculosis patient ward. In 1931, there was a second building, number 25, identical to the men's T.B. unit, that was built to house the Ladies' T.B. Unit. These two buildings were long sought for the hospital, as prior to their conception patients were just placed together regardless of health problem.

The census count on these units usually ran from 50-60 patients. In later years, when another building, number 33, was constructed, both men and women T.B. patients were housed in that unit. This in dormitory style. Continuing on with the south side, the next building was cottage 34. This cottage was built due south of cottage 32, some 60 feet away. This was a two story building, dormitory style rooms, with a few single bedrooms, which housed male patients who worked in the barn areas, as well as the kitchens and maintenance buildings. This cottage also was known as an open cottage, a designation that meant unlocked doors, no barred windows, and a good class of patients, some of whom worked in the greenhouse and garden areas.

The next building, and final one, was cottage 36. This unit also housed the workers' group. These men were usually in group labor activities in the farm field areas. This was a two story unit, which housed approximately 80-90 patients. The women's cottages were pretty much identical in size and structure. They usually housed some 40-50 people. Most were capable of working in maintenance areas, such as kitchens, sewing rooms and repair areas. The occupational therapy unit was usually comprised of groups of patients from many different areas.

Cottage 35 was built in 1932 and was a four-story building that housed bed-ridden patients. In 1937, now as an employee, I witnessed the construction of a four-story Receiving Building. Other than the original Building 50, this was the largest unit on the grounds. I was fascinated by all this growth, the labor was done by the patients, under supervision as well as other by skilled employees.

Building 50 was constructed totally of brick. Wood was used for roof supports and flooring. The lumber was garnered from nearby forests and was hard maple, beech and pine. If one could enter the attic areas, they would be awe-stricken by the size of the rafters which were 2'x6'. The number of bricks used in Building 50 alone have been estimated at 15 million. Both interior and exterior walls are five bricks wide, and laid side by side. The basement walls were of cut stone and shipped by sail boat primarily from Wisconsin, and the bricks were made on the shores of Cedar Lake. The enormous amount of brick helped to fashion the exterior walls that are still so beautiful.

The interior décor in building 50 was wood, the flooring was hard maple. Casements, arched doorways, wainscoting, cabinets and shelves were of basswood pine and even birch. The inner walls were plaster coated over the brick. Heating of the building was steam radiation, supplied from the power plant via tunnel and piping. Food was supplied from a central kitchen in the center of Building 50 and was taken through tunnels by rail carts to individual dining areas.

A question often asked is why building 50 and adjacent buildings were given numbers to designate them. In the beginning years, the buildings were assigned alphabetical letters. As the hospital grew and expanded, it was clear that the alphabet was not long enough to label all the buildings. At that time the hospital switched to a numerical system. With this system, it became labeled Building 50. The numbering was vital as far as identification in times of safety and emergencies. Later in the 1970s, patient and employee numbers were much lower than they had been, so additional numbering was added to maintenance structures in order to aid in fire protection duties.

The business offices were housed in Building 50 and were known as Center. This was the entry way to medical offices, which employed seven physicians when fully staffed. I only wish I could describe the beautiful woodwork that fashioned the walls, staircases, railings, etc. In 1959, all this section of Building 50 went under demolition and was replaced by a two-story building that for a short time was a nurses school. The former medical offices and business office were moved to a more advanced unit near the Receiving Hospital.

1934-1938

In February 1934, my father's health began to fail. He was 72-years-old and knew that something wasn't right. It wasn't until June that he was diagnosed with cancer. Surgery was performed in Ann Arbor, but, it was too late, which marked a drastic change in the Steele lifestyle.

Following his diagnosis of cancer, the hospital officials in Traverse City were of great help to us. When my father first became too ill to work, an agreement was reached that because of the knowledge I had of what was required in working in the greenhouse and garden areas, they would allow me to work as the assistant in that area. This would allow my father's paycheck to continue until such time as he could return to work.

This was accomplished through the auspices of Dr. Sheets, who was superintendent at that time. I will always be indebted to his compassion. He did much for my family and for me. as Dr. Sheets knew that my father was in terminal stages of cancer and was thinking in terms of our family's future.

In retrospect, I realize they knew that my father's condition was terminal and offered me employment to help us out, something that was accomplished prior to Civil Service in the State of Michigan departments came into effect. Had this happened within Civil Service, I, perhaps, would not have been offered the job.

This is a time in my life that I am ashamed to relay mostly with regards to helping my mother during her time of grief and change in lifestyle. During the six months prior to my father's passing, when I filled in at the greenhouse I was not, shall we say, a model employee. I shall always be amazed that they tolerated my behavior. The reason for my working in the greenhouse was to keep my father's paycheck coming in. In retrospect, this was not the happiest six-month period of my life. I was in a place that I didn't necessarily desire to be and did not draw any pay. My parents were in Ann Arbor, seeking treatment for my father's cancer. I lived in our hospital residence and took my meals along with the other employees in the kitchen nearest to my workstation, so although the hospital time sheets record the start of my employment with the hospital as being December 14, 1934, I must reaffirm that it actually started six months earlier.

While I was 19-years-old and should have had some beginning commitment to adulthood, I was still more the irresponsible teenager. My attitude provided many a headache to the assistant gardener. I know I festered a rebellious attitude rebelling often when asked to do something. Working hours were 7 a.m. until 5 p.m. with one hour for lunch and only every other Sunday off. With my mother and father in Ann Arbor, I was left home alone. I'd sometimes go to work at 10:00 a.m., maybe not until noon and the Sunday work-forget it! More often than not getting to work, I would just sit around. My boss was a great guy, but not given to being my boss, I took every advantage of him. He was an Englishman by nationality and a bachelor who actually started work at the hospital two years prior to my father in 1921 and passed away in 1941. Why he never reported my negligence, I'll never know.

I look back and think that I could have been more a companion and help to my mother. This is not to dismiss my father's input in my upbringing because he did influence a lot of happenings, even more after he had passed away. My parents were into middle age when I was born in 1914. My father was 54 and my mother was 31. Because I was an only child, much of what I learned was from them.

My father passed away on December 2, 1934. Services were held in Grand Rapids. With it being winter, travel was accomplished via railroad.

I think I shall always remember that trip coming back to Traverse City from Grand Rapids. It was so like the journey my mother and I had made some ten years prior on that snowy March evening. The night travel, coupled with the fact that we left behind our relatives in Grand Rapids, made mother and me realize that we were alone and not at all sure of our future. Coming into Traverse City late at night, we were met by friends who would have it no other way than having us stay with them until our immediate future was established. For that, I will always be thankful.

We had it quite easy during those years from 1923-1934, in that we were living in a furnished house. By this, I mean utilities, lights, heat and water were all furnished courtesy of the hospital. We did have our own furniture, and any furniture items we didn't own were on loan, again courtesy of the hospital. My father's compensation was based on housing and a $25.00 per month food supplement, again furnished by the hospital. For example, a loaf of bread was two cents. With my father in charge, we never lacked for vegetables. Our main grocery purchases were baked goods, meat, milk and eggs. We purchased, downtown, those items that the hospital did not stock. My father's paycheck was $100 a month, and he, while not a spendthrift, was rather loath to keep a savings account, so financial affairs were pretty much conducted "out of pocket." In their lifetime, they had three cars, which was a large portion of their financial expenditures. I never knew what was paid out for the first two cars owned. I knew that they were used cars, so probably not too great a cost. The third car, on the other hand, a 1929 REO Flying Cloud was purchased new. That nearly proved to be their financial undoing. At that time, October 1929, it would have qualified today as a big Buick or perhaps a small Cadillac. While the early payments "floored" them for awhile, they finally owned it-sadly, only a short while prior to Dad's passing. Looking back, I can only say I'm so very glad that they did have the pleasure of its use as both Mother and Dad had few pleasures.

The date was December 12, 1934. Mother and I went up to the hospital offices to find out what was to be in immediate effect. Speaking with the hospital business executive, Mr. Crawford, I was offered the assistant gardener's position. The former holder of that position had moved up into my father's position, which was only right. My mother asked, knowing that it probably couldn't be done, if we could stay in the housing that we had occupied for some ten years. The answer was "Sorry, no, it is part of the compensation for the head florist."

The new head gardener had his own home downtown and mandated that he did not wish to move to the grounds. In spite of this, we were forced to move and it is ironic that our home on the grounds remained empty for a matter of three years.

So with this edict and the request that we vacate by January 15, our first urgency was to relocate downtown. This duty fell upon my mother, as I had to start work immediately and as a new employee, had no leave-time coming. We found an apartment just off the hospital grounds on 11th Street, which allowed me to walk to and from work.

My wages were $85 a month take-home, the balances of compensation being room and board. I accepted the board, but tried to turn the "room" part into an additional amount on my check, which was met with "Sorry, take it or leave it." In those days, that were still considered "depression" days, one didn't argue with what they wanted, but simply took what was offered.

My mother had primarily been a homemaker for the ten years we resided in Traverse City, so she was at a disadvantage in seeking lodging off the grounds. The fact that it was mid-winter meant very little available housing. This did nothing to help the transition. It was through friends that we were finally able to secure our apartment on 11th Street. How well I remember the 7:00 a.m.-5:00 p.m. work hours. This time meant no skipping work in exchange for my own pleasure. I opted to accept the board and therefore ate my meals at the hospital. In order to have breakfast at the hospital, I had to be up at 5:00 a.m. in order to make the half-hour walk from our apartment to the hospital dining room. We had to place most of our household goods in storage as we were in a furnished apartment. Sadly, though, through poor security of the storage building, over the next few years we lost much of our more treasured items to theft.

In bleak wintertime, going to work at 7:00 a.m. and returning home at 5:00 p.m. meant arriving and leaving in the dark, because daylight did not occur until approximately 8:30 a.m. While the greenhouses were lit, it was of minimal effect, so work didn't start until sufficient daylight occurred. This brought about the first contradictory element between my boss and me.

I should explain my workstation and what it entailed. The original greenhouse, first constructed in 1892, consisted of four-80 foot long glass enclosed houses. An additional house was built in 1902. The mandatory need for food supplies, particularly fruits and vegetables, deemed it necessary to have some place to start a young seedling prior to outdoor field plantings. In the beginning the greenhouses were only used in the early spring months, but Dr. Munson, decided that it was wasteful in concept to use it only two months each year and that the balance of time the greenhouse would be used to raise floral items for ward decor within the hospital. This lead to additional houses being added on. The original greenhouses were primitive in concept with dirt floors, wooden benches, a cantankerous heating plant and a poor ventilation system.

In the late fall of 1933 until mid-summer of 1934, a new greenhouse was in the process of construction to replace the original structure, which was in ill repair and had little value. It had long been the desire of my father to have a new greenhouse complex constructed to his design, with a waist-high bench system. In early 1933, with the knowledge that a new greenhouse was to be built, my father was asked by the hospital business executive to contribute to the design. My father knew that I had exhibited some artistic talent, so he asked me to help in drawing up the desired design, which were then accepted by the business executive and given to the hospital maintenance supervisor, who put them into effect.

Upon completion, the greenhouse became the envy of commercial florists for miles around. Cement walks in all four houses, cement benches, and a raised heat source from the main power plant with a thermostatic control were just a few of the amenities.

One would have to work with, or at least be familiar with what greenhouse cultures consisted of in order to appreciate this modern structure, the epitome of design excellence. My father lived to see its completion, but never had the opportunity to work in or supervise the work within it. Fortunately, this is where I started.

There were four individual greenhouses. From late spring to early fall, two houses were given to raising head lettuce and radishes. From March until August, these houses were turned over to the raising of tomatoes and cucumbers. The remaining two houses were used for floral cultivation. These items were utilized in the ward living room decor as well as in Sunday chapel service. The floral content consisted of carnations, snapdragons, roses, chrysanthemum, plus many, many potted plant varieties. A very large outdoors-floral garden added additional floral beauty in the wards during the summer months. The floral line consisted of some 5,000 geraniums, 200 flats or boxes of petunias and many other summer florals.

There was little time for lax behavior. In the beginning months I was, through exposure over the years when Dad was in supervision, aware of the work ethics that were involved. In retrospect, though, I never thought all of this would constitute my life's endeavor.

The greenhouse was in use year round, dealing with the present harvest season and readying for the next. I came more in more direct contact with the patient personnel in small and large groups. There were three employees in the greenhouse department, which included the boss, myself and the outdoor gardener who, in the wintertime, oversaw the storage areas. Working within the greenhouse was a crew of five patients, all of whom were men, although in later years we had some women working in there, as well. The larger crews who were working in planting cultivation and harvest times could number as high as 90. In harvest season, we would see up to 60 women assistants in the small berry and cherry harvest. In early times, and even in times of my employment, this was a planned program of volunteer work therapy. if a negative response was made, the patient was asked to go out to the field area merely to get out of doors and sit on the edge of the work area. Invariably, after watching for awhile, they would voluntarily join in, which usually brought about a cheerful response to further work programming.

In the greenhouse work area, we had a crew of five resident workers. To verify the nationalities present at the hospital, of these five men, one was Polish, one Norwegian, one Hungarian, one Austrian and one German. As time went along and some of this conglomerate left, we had various other nationalities within the work force. All of the residents that I worked with were cooperative, rather than combative.

The resident labor assignments included an individual greenhouse to maintain, with plant care, watering, feeding and weeding. Transplanting and harvesting required assistance, and all of this was under the constant supervision of the Head Florist and me. When daily care in greenhouse areas was completed, the patients usually helped in the area we called a Service Room, where thousands of young seedling plants were transplanted to individual cartons for future planting in field areas.

It was within my capacity of Supervisor that I became acquainted with these "resident" individuals, more as a friend than boss.

About the Patients

The area where I lived had no companions of my age. While townspeople tolerated the institution for the jobs it offered the community; it wasn't an area where they wanted their children to be. Fear is somehow the most common association of the general public regarding the mentally ill. Even now, the public doesn't understand that mental illness, by its sometimes eccentric behavior, leads society to not understand it and therefore fear it.

As a young boy, the patients treated me very well. I think this was due to the fact that many, if not most, of the residents had come from families themselves, so I was treated accordingly. Those who were mentally disturbed to a point that was antagonistic, I simply steered clear of.

Many perceptions of what the institution was like were based on fears and apprehension. These were, and even continue to be, founded by misconceptions fostered by movies and books showing and telling of murderous people. This was never the case in my years of association with residents on the grounds. In my working years, I never saw the violence that was promoted in lurid detail in film and books.

By coincidence, prior to moving to Traverse City we lived in Ann Arbor in an area near the University of Michigan Psychiatric Hospital. We would occasionally see "walking parties" that would pass by our home. If I happened to be out in the yard and saw or heard them coming, I would run into the house until they would pass by. I still cannot fathom where my fear came from. They were always well behaved, and while talkative, were never violent.

Possibly, my fears were promoted by comments made by my elders, which were often made in jest. In earlier time, mental health, presumably because so little was known about it and even less about treating it, led to what is a misnomer of "warehousing". The barred windows and locked doors gave mental hospitals the titles of prisons. These restrictions were a protective barrier to the patient as well as the communities in which they lived. Custodial care without treatment was wrong. A hospital's main endeavor was to cure the ill, but so little was known of mental illness that actual cures were not available. Some who were afflicted did gain recovery and leave, but most were not so greatly helped. Possibly just a rest away from problems at home gave them the ability to re-gain good mental balance.

The hospital in Traverse City, through the efforts of its superintendent (a more forward-looking doctor,) did much to correct some attitudes outside as well as within the hospital. In the beginning years the patients were of much older age which led to a different example of complex behavior. One must remember the patients in earlier times who were of older age and their cases were simply senility. Those of more recent time were incapacitated through a lifestyle that couldn't be coped with. Just prior to my retirement, we witnessed an influx of mental illness rendered through drug addiction. This group was composed mostly teenagers and those in their early 20s. The truly pathetic thing was in the burnout, which resulted in "no way back" treatment. The patients of the 1920s and 30s were more amicable to work with. Some provided amusement through their hallucinations, such as imagining they were someone else. As a child exposed to this, I would sometimes wonder why, but as I grew older, the reason seemed to be that this was an escape method to get out of what was and return to another realm where their imagined greatness gave a feeling of a worthy life.

I recall such patients who gave way to their imaginative states. There was one who terrified me, momentarily at least, at age ten. Passing by where there was a laboring group, he suddenly grabbed me by the shoulders and started what I can only describe as an "Indian war dance." Muttering some unintelligible things, I struggled to escape. He finally stopped his motion and exclaimed, "Boy, how can I give you the powers if you won't stand still?" This caused much mirth on the part of the attendant guard who was standing nearby. You would have to personally witness this individual to appreciate his eccentricity. He imagined that he was King Tut of Egypt. He was some 65 years old and 200 pounds, wore a gray beard, and while his clothing was all intact, there were no areas anywhere that were not fastened with safety pins. He had necklaces of them all pinned together.

Another individual, a male quartered on the men's TB ward, sat out on a screened in porch and madly rocked away in a squeaking rocking chair. He imagined that he was God and gave forth in a loud voice the orders of what was to be done all over the earth on that particular day. It was fascinating to listen to as a young boy!

Another chap, was in his mind, a billionaire many times over, because he was determined to have and run a cookie factory. In this factory, the cookie would be frosted with gold dust and, of course, they would be free.

One middle-aged man, in remission in the TB ward, had gained ground parole. Everyday he would go to a water reservoir where the surplus water would cascade over a spillway some 18 feet in height. The man would disrobe and stand beneath the waterfall. The astounding part of this procedure was that he accomplished it on a daily basis, which meant winter and summer, from sub-zero temperatures to 80-degree weather, when the thermometer hovered around zero, the exclamations could be heard a mile away as he crawled beneath the icy waters, yet he always accomplished his task.

Strangely it seems that most of the more bizarre patients and activities embraced the male sector. I can't recall any women believing to be someone else, but in times of acute mental distress, they could put a sailor to shame with their use of profanity. My experience as a youngster of nine or ten was to steer clear of any area where a group of lady patients might be gathered. Insanity never affected their maternal instincts. Due to incarceration, they were starved of lavishing affection on children, so if I got near them I would be smothered with affectionate hugs and kisses. I learned quickly to be elsewhere when a group of women patients was passing by.

For the most part, I was living alone on the grounds in that there were no other boys around and the farm manager's daughters were not given outdoor privileges. There was a patient of the institution who had been a civil engineer. He ultimately succumbed to manic depression, and landed in the hospital where he stayed until he passed away. This was one of the tragedies in that he was one of a very few over all the years of my association who did commit suicide. His method was grim, although effective: he walked down the spur supply railroad track to the other main line going out of town. When the noon train came, he lay down on the tracks.

I had known this gentlemen only through brief meetings. He had worked as a parole patient with good sense in the hospital warehouse. Working in this area he had available to him scrap material, with which he constructed and gave to me homemade skis. These were made from barrel stave material with a leather thong for a footstrap. A barrel stave is a slightly curved piece of wood which, when brought together with several others with a ring type band, will form the sides of a barrel. Being that a stave has a slight curve to each end it presented a challenge as related to skiing dexterity, but they did prove entertaining. This same patient also made a toboggan for me, which I kept for years. In spring and summer he provided me with many different kites. He was quite a guy. I only wish that I could have realized a friendship with him that might have deterred him from suicide. But alas, I was only 12 when I knew him.

During this time I became very interested in trout fishing through the urging of another patient acquaintance. This man was a banking executive who fell upon hard times by way of his fraudulent banking practices. His choice was either Jackson prison or the Traverse City State Hospital. I never saw him do anything unusual (as might occur from a mentally ill standpoint), and we became quite good friends. In my youth, he taught me a lot of what is known today as environmental process. This included knowledge of fishing and picking of berries and fruits in the wilderness areas.

One day while stream fishing I ran into another patient who was also fishing. Noting some clumsiness on my part with regard to technique, he volunteered to help me out. About a week later, I went stream fishing with him again. On about my third fishing trip with him, my father took note and told me, "I do not want you to go with him." I questioned why, but my father simply responded, "Never mind, just don't go."

With that wording, I consequently did as I was told. In later conversation with my mother, I made mention of my father's restriction. She was surprised that he hadn't told me his reasoning. The patient, when a member of society, was a farmer in the Mt. Pleasant area. One summer day he accompanied his nine-year-old son who was bringing a load of hay into the barn from the field. Riding atop the hay load, the boy was munching on an apple and mischievously threw the core so that it hit one of the horses. The horse became spooked and led the team into running away. This resulted in the ultimate overturning of the wagon and throwing both the father and son to the ground. The father recovering first saw his son lying on the ground. The father, enraged because of the accident, picked up a wood splinter from the wagon wreckage and stabbed his son to death. This made very clear my father's reasoning.

This next story involves a resident not working in the greenhouse, but rather a visitor there. He was a kindly 80-year-old retired lawyer, experiencing the beginning of senility; alert, but at the same time fading. His professional career had been spent in Chicago and it was fascinating to hear his tales of the big city.

As a widower he established a home with his daughter in Ludington. His daughter, a graduate of Wellesley College and quite wealthy, brought him to live with her as he began showing his disability. Eventually, she placed him in our hospital. In gaining ground parole and using the greenhouse and ultimately becoming friendly with me, he found me to be a sympathetic listener. He finally asked me if I would bring him a daily Chicago Tribune to read. Because he was buying, I suggested that while I was more than willing to pick it up for him, he could achieve the same through the mail office of the hospital. This was one of the odd behaviors he displayed, trusting no one in an official position, so I started serving as paper boy for him, which led to a more serious problem. One day I brought my still camera to work to take some pictures of the greenhouse. These were to be entirely unrelated to residents, as it was a strict no-no to ever take any photographs of them.

He happened to see my camera and begged me to take some pictures for him to give to his daughter who visited frequently. When I commented that it was forbidden, he said they were not to be pictures of him. He wanted pictures of the grounds that he liked. I told him "we'll see," hoping that in a few days the whole thing would be forgotten. He badgered me to get some film and have it processed at his expense. Finally I agreed, obtained the film and started out on the grounds snapping pictures of the areas he designated, making sure that he was never within the camera lens. This went on for two or three shootings. I was getting more uncomfortable in doing so, and finally decided to firmly tell him "no more." My mistake was in not ceasing earlier or perhaps in doing it at all. For the last roll we ascended a high hill to the rear of the grounds called Pikes Peak which had a panoramic view of the bays. In order to get all of this in I had to take several pictures that when developed and laid side-by-side would offer a panoramic view of Traverse City from Marion Island to the distance south. Our resident friend proclaimed this to be the final series he desired. A few days after the prints were obtained, I was summoned at work by phone call. The caller was the local FBI agent who asked, who the hell I thought I was taking these pictures? When I related I was only doing this as a goodwill gesture to a resident, he demanded to know who the resident was. When I said that such information would have to be obtained through hospital officials, he calmed down, thanked me and said he would get back to me. Very shortly, I received another phone call from hospital officials, blistering me for my violation of the "no photographs" rule.

Now to explain the violation that involved the FBI. It was mid 1942, we were at war and the Navy had taken over the airport here as a naval air station. The FBI had instigated a program with local film processors to be notified of any film they developed which showed up suspicious in local views. It seems my panoramic view of Traverse City, inclusive of the airport to the East, intrigued the FBI to no end. With this episode, I resolved and stuck to it that my good will gestures were limited to conversation only.

The following may seem to demonstrate conceit, but it is not intended. It is merely to demonstrate what I felt, and what I did for resident welfare with regard to work areas. Somewhere along the early 1960s, I knew the hospital was giving a party that included a luncheon and entertainment. Award certificates were handed out to employees for services above and beyond the call of duty with regards to the residents. Going to this party, I fully expected the certificate awards would deal in direct areas where personnel interacted with residents. The State Mental Health Director was a guest at this luncheon and he handed out the certificates in the hospital's large auditorium, which could hold some 300 employees. I was called up to the stage area three times to receive these commendations. I was embarrassed the first time up, so you can well imagine how I felt on the second and third call. This was because I was aware of others, such as nurses and social workers, who worked more closely with greater groups of residents and knew these people were not happy with one person receiving three awards. I was proud and flattered to be honored for something I did out of consideration from one human being to another. It was a rather unwritten rule that an employee be respectful of a resident and his particular mental problem.

Part of dealing with the residents was to be sympathetic and understanding of their problems, but, more importantly, to be aware that there were those who would also take advantage of the sympathy offered. How well I learned this latter concept when I let my judgment lapse. One example proved to be more devastating in outcome to the resident than it did to me.

This resident approached me one Saturday at the greenhouse and begged me to help him write a letter to his girlfriend beseeching her to come and visit. Not having much to do and being alone, I agreed. After telling me the situation with his girlfriend, it was his desire that I tell him what to write. They both lived in West Branch, which was not that far from the hospital. The letter was formulated and duly dispatched. Two weeks later, again on a Saturday, he approached me. He was very agitated to the point of throwing himself into the nearest river. What he told me this time, had been left out of our prior conversation. This gentleman was a 50-year-old man, married and an alcoholic, with a girlfriend on the side. When his wife discovered his philandering, she had herself appointed as his guardian and brought him to the institution to cure his alcoholism. I had not known that he had written to his wife begging her to come see him. He told her that he had been cured and he would never stray again. Receiving this letter and desiring to believe him, she did come for a visit that Saturday. The only problem was that the girlfriend, who was contacted via the letter, also came and arrived first, and they were together when the wife drove up to the cottage where he resided. When she recognized what was going on, she kept right on going. After the girlfriend departed, he came to the greenhouse very distraught. He knew he had thoroughly ruined his ability to persuade his wife to gain his release. To finalize the story she sent him a letter stating that she was returning to Texas, where they had originally come from. She was intent upon obtaining a divorce. She was terminating her guardianship and as far as she was concerned, he could "rot" in Traverse City for the rest of his life.

The final summation was that he showed her letter to his social service caseworker and as he was a resident case in alcoholic nature, he was released. That taught me a lesson in cooperating during a marital dispute. Fortunately none of this ever came to the attention of the hospital authorities or I could have gotten in trouble for meddling where I had no right to be.

Patient Lifestyles

With today's attitude about smoking in public areas, I am reminded of numerous times in the museum when I was often asked what was offered to the residents with regard to tobacco.

The residents were given, if they so desired, tobacco in all forms, in measured quantities, twice a week. The chewing tobacco was described as "plug." Smoking tobacco for pipe use and loose tobacco for "roll your own" cigarettes was provided. Most residents preferred the "roll your own" style and some were skilled in fashioning a roll. Many, however, were not that talented and the results were rather sad. There were restrictions on carrying lighting materials in early times. Any resident desiring to smoke had to go to a definite smoking room and have his "desire" lit by a ward employee, which often led to just giving up the smoking habit altogether.

What was interesting was how tobacco was handled. It was brought to the institution from State Department warehouses, sent to the hospital warehouse and then dispensed to individual wards or cottages who would place orders for their needs. The cut plug came in huge sheets, 30 by 40 inch size, to be exact. The hospital warehouse would cut this package to one by two inch squares and dispense it to the residents at their twice weekly request.

As one might suspect, the work involved to get to the point of actually smoking the tobacco product often deterred the patients from bothering in the first place, so there was less use than what was probably thought.

The women's area was extended the same courtesy, but was minimally used until smoking became more popular in the later years. The lighting of tobacco also meant that residents were free to carry matches. I can only recall one intentionally set fire. This occurred when a young woman, who was mentally retarded, became enraged when she was refused permission to smoke. She promptly raced to her room, went into her closet and attempted to set her room on fire. Luckily, another resident caught her in the act and promptly stopped her. As punishment, ground parole was denied for several days. To lose ground parole was a more fitting punishment than any other form, because it was a cherished privilege.

In the mid 1970s, the canteen was established providing all the more reason to want ground privileges. The canteen provided light lunches, coffee, pop, and the like, and writing materials were also available.

Another item that was a luxury, was something that was ongoing from the time I first arrived on the grounds. An enterprising young male resident fashioned a four wheeled manually powered cart with a canvas covered roof top, very reminiscent of a covered wagon. This man evidently had an ongoing arrangement with a wholesale grocery and supplied candy, cigarettes and other small salable items. On Sundays and holidays, he would start out with his wagon, traverse the grounds directly adjacent to the buildings and sell his goods. He only sold very small items, such as candy bars and they were very popular and their minimal size helped out. A good number of his customers were residents on second, third and fourth floor ward areas and this man was not allowed to enter the wards to conduct sales, so residents on the upper floor levels would use a small sack tied to a lengthy string and lower their coins to the ground. Their goods would then be sent back up in a similar fashion. All this was done on the honor system, but with the advent of the resident "canteen" his business promptly failed.

An interesting side note is how the holidays, specifically Thanksgiving, Christmas and Easter, were handled for the residents. There were other holidays of less interest, but nonetheless meaningful to the residents. The residents with relatives would receive gifts from home, but the reality existed that many residents were elderly men with no relatives living.

Dr. Munson and his Dietary department did go all out with food festivities. They also had church services, with ministers coming in to conduct services in the Chapel Room in Building 50. Incidentally Dr. Munson was adamant that all residents capable of attending Church were required to do so.

In later years, residents were encouraged to go home for the holidays, if their mental state would allow that opportunity. Many times, the patient was approved to go home, but the family refused to let them come. Officials involved in visitation rights always had to affirm that the resident would be welcome. Many residents left at the Hospital, went into depression, while some others entered into periods of violence. For the most part, they eventually recovered. Many residents, who were rejected by their families were for the most part alcoholics or mentally unfit. Those residents remaining were given additional attention in a social time with dances, cards parties and gifts.

In the early 1960's more public attention was given to the needs of the residents not just at holiday time, but year-around. Ohmer Curtis was appointed as a Community Relations Officer and he was a very capable person, as well as a minister in church areas.

He immediately started corresponding with church memberships, social clubs and social groups, asking these groups, to please send suitable small gift items to the Hospital to be properly wrapped and then dispensed to the residents. This correspondence was sent to all 39 counties which the Hospital served.

Mr. Curtis, had crossed his fingers in hopes that he might receive some help, but he had no idea the immense return mail that he would ultimately receive. There was so much so that I was drafted from the Greenhouse to assist in unloading huge cartons of gifts to be cataloged and thanked for later.

The gifts were sent to volunteer groups to be wrapped, and on Christmas Day, they were given to the residents. This was the method where the holiday was brought home to the resident, along with gifts from their family, church services, special dinners served by the Dietary Department and a special New Year's Eve dancing party put on by the employees.

This entertainment went on annually through the 1960's and 1970's and until the hospital closed 1989. I participated voluntarily in most of these events. The enjoyment I derived was that in participation, the residents recognized you were helping them celebrate.

Other events that residents could enjoy, under supervision, were attending traveling circuses that came to town annually, The Northwestern Fair in the fall, and especially the 4th of July with a big picnic, sponsored by the Hospital. The National Cherry Festival came later, but was eagerly attended by residents who relished attending the parades.

A Recreation Department was finally established to cover the increasing needs in this area, and it was staffed by trained personnel. Entertainment activities became a weekly event, music was taught to residents, and eventually, an orchestra was formed to entertain at party events. Classes in art were also common.

In the 1950's, the Hospital purchased an acreage on West Bay for a picnic grounds for the residents. All departments contributed to the improvements of the grounds and the construction of a "changing-house". Picnics were held there until the Hospital closed, at which time the property was donated to the Bingham township.

I often think that people passing by the Hospital wondered what the residents did. Did they sit in chairs and do nothing? Actually they participated in some activity, be it work by choice, learning by choice or at other times entertainment.

The patients in the work force were housed separately from the main group. These buildings or dormitories were called open wards, which meant unlocked doors at all times and unbarred windows. These buildings housed 60-80 patients and because of their freedom, were desirable housing.

In earlier times, when therapeutic measures were minimal, these people could well spend most of their lives in this particular element. As psychoanalysis and chemotherapy became more prevalent, their stays were minimal. They were usually kept to working class status to avoid contact with the more unruly patients and disrupt treatment. This is not to say that they were the only ones receiving attention, only that they were nearer to a return to society.

In the institution's beginning, many of the patients were middle-aged to elderly. Most were in poor physical health and many were mentally disabled. Many were lumberjacks who had come to the end of their careers, and the medical policy at this time was to respond to their physical needs and prepare them to comprehend that this would be their final home.

There was another category of patients-those who were foreign born. Most came to this country in high hopes of a future, but invariably they were poorly educated and brought no particular work skills, which ultimately led to nervous breakdowns and eventually to institutionalization.

The hospital was not off limits to the well-to-do or well-educated members of society.

The female population of the hospital consisted primarily of farm wives who were overburdened with work, childbearing and poor economic standards. Most had suffered nervous breakdowns. Scattered among the preceding were those who were mentally retarded and, until legislative amendment prohibited, a group of grandpas and grandmas showing signs of senility, what we probably know to be Alzheimer's

Disease. Family members who were eager to be rid of the responsibility of home care often shoved these older folk into the institution. In my past meetings with the public as museum curator, a commonly asked question was "Wasn't that a dominant factor even in more recent times?" I would reply that law prohibited it, the answer I think they desired. Even today, there is a misconception which I certainly witnessed during my 50 years of exposure to mental health- the idea that the mentally ill were violent to the point of criminal behavior was not so in the main group. Invariably, mental breakdown brought out peculiarities of action. Public awareness of this promoted a misunderstanding, which in turn brought about the worst case scenario, and all of this brought difficult times to patients whom recovered, but found it difficult to gain a re-acceptance into society.

If a patient were to become unruly within the institution, they were placed on a ward until they calmed down. Unfortunately, these wards were in an area where the general public would be aware of noise and activity and draw the conclusion that the institution was as a whole a violent place.

1939-1957

I was poorly prepared for management status, something I found out with my sudden exposure to management when the boss Alfred Leland suffered a kidney stone attack that took him out of the picture for a month during a crucial time during the spring. His absence necessitated doing reports that had to be sent to the business office on both a daily and monthly basis. This was accomplished with the aid of the third employee, who primarily conducted the supervision of vegetable storage areas and attended the plantings, and cultivation and harvesting in the spring, summer and early fall. With his help, we weathered the absence of the boss.

In 1939, I had to assume the same supervisory role, when Mr. Leland again became ill. This time it was a heart attack, which kept him away for two months in mid-summer. By this time, I was more familiar with what was mandatory as far as departmental bookkeeping. I make mention of this more because the "big boss" (the hospital business executive, that is) was somewhat difficult to work for in that he was an alcoholic and tended to be dictatorial in department management. His problem made it precarious to deal with him and I shall always suspect that the constant brow beating he was constantly administering caused the health problems that afflicted my boss, Mr. Leland, who took it and he didn't fight back. In later years this "big boss" tried it with me. I took it for awhile, but one day I blew back and it ceased.

My social life was fairly minimal. Shortly after graduating in 1933 from high school, I met a girl with whom I kept company until she graduated from high school in 1935. At that time she left town to seek her fortune in Detroit. She and her family were very supportive of my mother and myself in the month's following my father's death. They were very kind. I am still in contact with her and her husband.

Following her move to Detroit, I dated casually-nothing serious, though. In springtime 1939, I was introduced to Marion Mead, by a mutual friend. My first meeting with Marion could not exactly be called a date. Our mutual friend, Fitz, decided on a beautiful Easter Sunday to drive up to Mackinaw City for something to do. On our way out of town, he spotted Marion parking the family car, in front of her families' drugstore. He stopped momentarily to talk to her and invite her along to Mackinaw City. There began an intense campaign on my part to win her affection as she had several other suitors. There were stormy periods as well as great times during the holiday season of 1939-1940. I won out and we made plans for a June wedding.

In late spring 1938, I had become increasingly bored with my job at the hospital, but decided there was no other line of work in Traverse City, so I stayed at the hospital. In June, the state of Michigan assumed Civil Service for all state employees, which was meant to prevent large turnover of state employees each time there was gubernatorial election. Previously, with each party change in Lansing, there were subsequent down-the-line firing and replacement with party faithfuls.

The inception of Civil Service was feared and dreaded more specifically in my area of work. This was due to the fact that most employees in the farming area were uneducated and in my area, I was the only high school graduate.

In the beginning, Civil Service job testing was very simple. It was really merely a general test for all the employees with the intent that a more difficult exam was required for different departments. One employee who worked in the maintenance department area as a painter, held this position for many years and was really an expert in all categories of his job. He reckoned that having quit school in sixth grade, he didn't stand a chance in the "new wrinkle," Civil Service, so he refused to take the first exam and consequently had to resign. This happened in spite of his bosses, clear up to the superintendent, urging him to take the exam, all to no avail. Most of the early employees were dedicated to their duties, but for the most part lacked formal education. Still, they were all wonderful people and gave much of themselves in the area of patient care.

By 1936, my mother had recovered from her grief and had taken over the rooming house in which our apartment was located, but soon found she was not committed to being a landlord and gave up that position for duties as a clerical worker in a downtown store. By this time, family friends in Ann Arbor urged my mother to return, and even found a job for her as a housekeeper for a recently widowed young man with two small children. Thus, she moved from Traverse City, never to return other than for a visit.

In late 1939, having announced our intent to marry, I began seriously considering a change of job. While the job I took over in 1934 was still in existence, it had not produced anything in promotional or financial benefits. At this time, my mother was a housekeeper for a family who had close ties with the president of the Detroit Edison Company. In conversation, these friends learned that I was seeking to improve my work status. Through some string pulling, I gained an interview with the CEO of Detroit Edison in March of 1940. Out of this meeting came a request in early April to come to Detroit for another interview at a huge power plant called the Connors Creek Plant that serviced the Chrysler Car Company in that area of Detroit. My work would be a continuation of the field that I was presently working in, and would include ground maintenance, lawns, trees, shrubbery and floral bed maintenance. The Edison Plant had a huge grounds area all bordering the Detroit River, and I came away from this interview very assured that I'd soon be a "working stiff" in Detroit.

Coming back to Traverse City and knowing that I'd soon be moving away, I thought it best to relate my intent to the Superintendent of the hospital, the man who happened to be the benefactor of all my adult work years.

Before I could meet with him a series of events took place that as I look back now, I realize brought about the future and all that was for me for 50 years. Shortly after I returned to my workstation, awaiting notification from Detroit, I learned that my boss, Mr. Leland, had been stricken with a severe heart attack. He recovered, but it took him some three months to do so. Once again, this threw me into the "in charge" position.

At this time, the superintendent called me in to tell me of my duties. I relayed to him my intent with the Detroit venture. He was somewhat taken aback, but graciously accepted the fact that I desired to better my future and myself. He was very aware of the minimal wages paid to the agricultural department employees and explained to me that my leaving would certainly be a disadvantage to the hospital as we were well into the heavy spring program in gardening and were one man short in the department due to Mr. Leland's illness. Coming away from his office in a much-troubled state of mind, I was also aware that Marion had mentioned that perhaps we should wait to get married until I was sure of the possibility of Detroit. At this time, the thought of staying in Traverse City took root in a very foot firming way. In contemplation, I wondered if maybe this was where God wanted me. I've never, ever regretted the decision to stay.

I consequently notified all the necessary individuals and stayed on in Traverse City. Marion and I were married in June 1940. With the gracious kindness of her parents, we set up housekeeping in the upstairs at 620 State Street. Marion got a job in her family's drugstore, and I, remained on at the hospital. Soon after marriage, I sought some financial improvement in "take home" pay and did succeed in gaining back the deduction taken out for room and board. This brought the take home pay up from the original $85 a month to $110. At this time the hospital established a meal ticket method of meal purchase which helped quite a bit.

In September 1940, we discovered a child, whom we would name Ron, would join us in June 1941. With the excitement and anticipated joy came the determination to improve living and job conditions. In early 1941, I gained a promotion in job title which also produced an improvement in wages to $125 a month. Those were very good years though they contained minimal activity in social nature. Wartime commitment frugality, plus no transportation until 1945 eased this situation when we purchased a family car Marion's parents had owned.

In the continuing war years of 1945, our travels were minimal due to gas restrictions. After that, with the war over, we were able to do more distant traveling. In 1946, a daughter, Marilyn, joined us. In 1947, we sold the car as its maintenance costs were evermore increasing, and were without transportation until 1949, when we were able to purchase our first new car. Through the car-less times, I used local taxi service to get to work in the mornings and then walked home in the evenings.

In May 1941, Mr. Leland passed away with a fatal heart attack. This once again placed me in charge temporarily. As the dust settled in Mr. Leland's departure, the superintendent again called me into his office and told me of his great regret that he could not offer me the department superintendency because of State Civil Service requirements. It seemed that anyone seeking state employment was required to take an exam governing whatever area they desired. Through this exam medium, they would establish a bank of potential employees from which, in time of need, they would call upon. My error was that the exam governing my department area occurred when I was strongly intending to leave state service. I knew of the exam date, but didn't attempt to take it. Ironically, it would have shortened the procedure that I went through in following years.

Once again, I managed the greenhouse during its busiest season until they could establish who among the top three candidates would qualify and consequently be the boss. I was not bothered by having a stranger come in as a supervisor and in fact, I was looking forward to the succession in that I was weary of the struggle to maintain the quality we had when we operated at full force. It probably sounds a bit ludicrous that three employees could accomplish that much more than two, but while you had a work force of five steady, year round patient source labor groups, it would increase during planting, cultivation and harvest times to as many as 100 patients who demanded constant, and close, supervision because of mental attitude or lack of the same.

When the candidate came along, he just couldn't fathom my enthusiasm for the fact that he was there. In our first meeting and my detailing of duties and expectations, he kept saying, "This should be your job. You deserve it!" I didn't elaborate on why I was so pleased with his coming, for fear he wouldn't stay. It was August 1942 when this new boss, Mr. Burton Fry, took over. Fry was a Michigan State University graduate with a degree in horticulture. He came upon the scene a widower of 38 years who was originally from Lansing, MI. He had very little time to absorb duties in regards to his job when he was called to military duty in January 1943, leaving me in charge. This time, I benefited greatly in that I was promoted in job rank to Florist A from Florist B, again a requisite of Civil Service. In November 1945 Burton Fry, returned from his war service and I dropped back to the Assistant Florist rating. My tenure as boss was difficult because wartime curtailments in material requisitions and employee replacements provided many difficulties. In fact, from a normal three-employee group in the garden department no replacement for him was ever effected, leading to a thin spread of capabilities in necessary areas, with some disastrous results. Because I was in charge, even if only temporarily, I felt it reflected on me. Management never complained, but for me it was great relief to turn over the supervisory element.

My mother had a succession of jobs over the years from 1937-1948 and finally landed a job working at St. Joseph's Mercy Hospital. She worked in the housekeeping area until she became terminally ill in 1953, and passed away following a short illness. Ironically, she had undergone a mandatory physical exam required of all hospital employees and had passed with flying colors. She suffered a severe stroke two weeks later, lingered for nearly a week and then had a final stroke. She had been with us in Traverse City on vacation only a couple weeks before and to me she seemed to have never been in better health. With that in memory, we shall close out my time with my parents. We were a close family.

The years of 1945 through 1957 saw a pattern, then unsuspected, but one of long intent by Lansing directive—that being the ultimate closure of all farming activities at the institution. By 1950, we as employees held a growing suspicion that something was afoot. One would have to know of the intensity of production efforts over the many years in assistance of hospital costs, particularly in food production element. In the years of 1950-1957, when edicts from Lansing State Agricultural Department called for curtailments in production, the question was raised, as to what was happening.

We had all begun to suspect in the early 1950s that the hospital was in the early stages of closure. The many edicts coming forth from the Mental Health Department in Lansing pointed to down sizing, although it did take some 30 plus years to accomplish, in total, the closure. By 1989, the hospital was totally shut down.

In 1956, the ultimate became manifest with the total closure of the dairy department. February 1957 saw the sale of the dairy heard, some 400 head of prize Holstein cattle. After the more valuable cattle within the group had been dispersed to other institutions, the balance of some 100 cows were auctioned off to the public in an auction conducted on the grounds that brought prospective purchases from all over the nation and even Canada.

With the farm closed, a mandate was in need as to what to do with some 18 employees in that department. Those of us in the greenhouse area were so positive that we would be the first to go. The dairy dispersal brought the need for the sale of outlying farmlands that the dairy once needed in support areas, primarily hay, field corn, etc., and one closure prompted another. In January 1957, a need arose to do something with the employee roster.

This time became a time of dread for Burton Fry, myself and the third employee in our greenhouse. Our most needed area was that of starting, planting, cultivating and harvesting vegetables, realized with the loss of patient labor in 1957. Burton and I were sure that we would be closed out as well, but strangely again, the decision was rendered to keep the greenhouse.

At this point a meeting between employees and management officials brought decision time and produced relief for me as to the immediate future.

Hospital officials, of course, were required to dismiss the employees. State Civil Service mandated at that time that said employees be melded into other areas of the institution, including nursing, dietary, laundry, etc., where most of the farm employees went.

This resulted in the formation of a new department, the very one in which I completed my employment. The supervisor of this department had been the former farm manager and his assistant was the former dairy boss. I followed them in that I had garnered out of this department change a promotion to Groundsman A. It was a lowly title, but established in order to further eventual promotions. It provided a little difficulty for awhile with employees who at that time were lesser ranking titles with regards to Civil Service, and their anger was based partially in that prior to promotion, I had been in the same ranking. One or two of these were older in years than me, but not in hospital employment, and they were offended for awhile.

There has often been wonderment as to why a company or corporation would go outside of its own personnel to find someone to take over a position thought to be promotable within the organization. This is in contradiction to what happened for me. I would have been in favor of finding someone new to head the department. I had learned much on my way up the ladder. Having been one of the boys, I knew all the changes that took place when one became boss and I realized that trying to find a middle ground just didn't work favorable, as far as the success of the department. Fortunately, I had no enemies at that time. My feeling is that the department would have accomplished more if all feelings had been of mutual respect.

The new department was established to maintain the ground area primarily during the summer, with lawn mowing and maintaining trees, shrubbery and such floral décor as is still in existence. Winter work was more maintenance including snow removal from walks, roads and driveways. Service maintenance consisted of laundry trucks for delivering and picking up garbage and for general hauling of lumber.

With lawn maintenance being primarily of mowing detail, the institution was forced to buy mechanized equipment, because in the past the workload was handled by a patient crew of 30 or more patients. The original mechanization consisted of one large tractor. Over the next four years we purchased six more. I inherited the first tractor and operated it until a back injury surfaced and I couldn't ride it anymore, at which point I inherited a sub-department position that included tree and shrubbery maintenance. This was an area that I enjoyed immensely. The area is now long in need of care, but even yet, it is visible what benefits were derived. Wintertime duties, of course, were snow removal by way of heavy equipment used to clear roads, parking lots and sidewalks.

And so passed the 1950s.

1960 and Beyond

The next change for me came in 1967 when, through the retirement of the assistant supervisor of the department, I was promoted to that position. The only difference in work was that it involved more paperwork and supervisory duties in the absence of the department superintendent.

Here again, friction arose because of a youngster being boss. Strangely, and somewhat satisfyingly, as these old employees took retirement, they would approach me and apologize for their attitudes. It didn't really bother me too much other than when it occasionally disrupted department harmony and task accomplishment. Little did I know what the future would have in store for me within the department.

My responsibilities stayed the same until 1972 when the department superintendent retired and I came into full charge, effective October 1, 1972

This promotion had a strange element with regards to civil service. With the formation of the grounds department in 1957, department head was given the civil service classification of farm manager 9. The transfer from farm manager 9 to ground supervisor 9 wreaked havoc in grounds department circles with regards to other institutional areas. This was due to the only other superintendent 9 being the man in charge of the state Capitol area grounds. This somehow passed seemingly unnoticed by civil service officials, and when it did come to light, it caused much friction for them. They vowed that with the next person to be promoted, the problem would be corrected, meaning the position would be de-classified to the next lower level which happened indeed.

The proceeding did effect the level at which I completed my final years of service. I was entitled as a superintendent eight. I didn't resent this lower-level in that I knew I was entering my final work years and to enter into legal protest would undoubtedly have taken a good many years and I would have been at the seven level and lost out on the compensation features of an 8. This related to the final computation for pension benefits.

With the ascension to department head, it lessened field activity for me and added on more office work. I started out in the field directly after assuming the department head only to incur the wrath of my boss, who could never reach me in the office. He strongly told me to stay put in the office area, and I did so, albeit reluctantly. It was boring being held to my office rather supervising the field. The one benefit early enjoyed from this new prominence was to have a department pickup truck to get around in.

With all of this going on, the hospital continued in the direction of the move toward closure. In mid 1957 we saw the installation of mental health treatment methods that were astounding in that both long and short-term patients responded quickly and could leave the institution. They were not necessarily cured but were able to return to society. With a census of 3600 in 1960, this number dropped by the hundreds in the ensuing years. With this trend, many wards were combined and some closed totally. Once again the question of "what do we do with the employee personnel?" arose. Some filled positions in other departments where retirement of personnel had occurred. This came about in my department in that I had employees who had either reached mandatory retirement age of 70 or had elected to go sooner.

It fell into my lap to interview and decide who among the lay offs was best suited to enter my department and there is no quicker method to make enemies or friends for that matter! I was ultimately about 98% successful in gaining good help. The 2% were somewhat of a headache during a rest of my tenure. By now, my department, by adding responsibilities in the transportation department, had grown to 10 employees. With the ever growing number of lay offs in nursing and dietary departments, my own group became more and more disgruntled and worried as to how long it would be before it was them.

In 1976, I received another added department through the retirement of a department head. This group was called Labor crew and its origination had taken on the duties formerly performed by patient workgroups. These personnel totaled some eight employees. Through office edict, they came from other departments such as dietary. They were disgruntled by lay offs within the kitchen because work in my department earned less pay and seemingly more work.

In 1976, change was affected in department directors, consolidation being a more apt description. I found myself again with a new boss, with whom I had been the best of friends. When he came out of the ranks and took charge of this department, carpentry maintenance, he became impossible to get along with. He had come up through the work crew in the carpenter shop area. While best friends with this worker at that time, when he became a supervisor, he was despised. With turning the Labor crew over to me from his charge, he immediately set up a new office for me adjacent to his. This enraged my original crew in that they had to report to me in a different location, so these became the most difficult years my tenure of service. This was from 1976 until 1980 when this boss suffered a heart attack and had to retire. He passed away two years later.

Now we approach the beginning times that brought about my retirement years- specifically the museum. In 1978, I was put in charge of procuring storage for many artifacts that had been in a jumble in one of the closed buildings. No particular security meant that many of the more valuable items were lost or stolen. I requested and received permission to set up a display element. In early stages, this did not attract much attention, but it did effect more security and did bring about visitation in the ensuing years.

1984 brought the conclusion of my employment. I could have retired in 1979, being at that time 65 and eligible for Social Security, but Marion still desired to continue on in her work, so I decided to stay on until the state mandatory retirement was effective, 70 years of age.

They were all good years. Many friends were made, and always the most gratifying was the extended show of friendliness. This was exhibited at the hospital retirement party when hospital employees still working as well as many that had retired came forth to wish me well. And even today in chance meetings in malls or restaurants, some will call me by name. More often than not I don't know them, but only surmise that they worked somewhere in the institution.

Another pleasing element, albeit a sad one is that many coworkers have gone down the road, but many still remember me on sight and make known times gone by. I am saddened by the deterioration that is now ongoing, and I can hardly describe my feelings viewing the deterioration of what was so beautifully rendered for the mentally ill over those early years.

Post-retirement

This time period embraces my efforts and those of my associate retiree personnel in the establishment improvement, and publicity of the museum.

Some early post-retirement era functions included the honors I received in a Lansing meeting in June 1984 for some 50 years of service to the State Mental Health Department, represented by then Gov. Jim Blanchard; Director of Mental Health Department Patrick Babcock, State Senator Mitch Irwin and State Representative Tom Power.

The early beginnings of the museum were in 1950, when its first conception came from a man by the name of Chet Krum. He was a former nursing supervisor who inherited (by state fire marshal office) the task of removing from various building attics artifacts now to be seen in the museum. Its beginnings were small and seldom seen by the public, and a few years later, they were removed from display area for needed space. This is when I came upon the scene. My involvement consisted of removing items and placing them to a sufficient storage area until proper housing for a museum could be found. While doing this, I thought it would be nice if more items in other areas could be brought together and restored to proper exhibit form.

I was to find proper storage for such items, and any items that I couldn't find storage for, I was to destroy. The collection had grown in size and value, so I quickly found temporary storage, but I soon discovered that the area had no security and some of the valuable items were disappearing. Once again, I went in search of a more secure building and permission to use it. As time would allow, I started assembling and arranging artifacts that I felt were worthy to be displayed. Tight security was maintained and hospital officials would visit the "museum" from time to time. They became enthused and put me in charge of the museum when the public would visit.

When I attained the required retirement age in 1984, I was asked to voluntarily maintain the museum, and said yes. Other retirees, as well as employed personnel joined in to help. The museum was growing in size and quantity and was becoming a very popular place to visit.

In those retirement years, and with the aid of fellow retirees, the artifact exhibit took on a professional appearance, which lead to a museum association being established to preserve and maintain the collection. With the total closure of the hospital, the museum fell upon hard times, even though we did inherit many objects of antiquity, enough to fill another building. In only three years of daily opening, we had nearly 8000 people visit. The value of the artifacts has been assessed at $200,000!

Unfortunately, our joy and pleasure was short lived. The museum relied on the institution remaining open, but as of October 1, 1989 the institution was closed, thus ending the museum's "life."

My fear was that the general public would be robbed the first-hand knowledge of what elements were involved in early mental health treatment and facilities, a fear validated when items from the hospital went on the auction block during the summer of 1998. There was a local historical association that was very interested in taking over managing its future, but with little finance and political clout, it never worked out.

At this time, the Archives Department of the Michigan State museum in Lansing came and garnered a great deal of the collection. With the buildings and grounds being sold privately, a general sale was held, and the local historical society did gain some artifacts.

While there were many humorous times throughout the years, there were also tragic and pathetic elements as well. In the beginning, the greenhouse in which I labored year round had a year round patient crew of five men who varied in intelligence from engineers with college educations to dropouts with some degree of retardation. In the course of the years in association with the hospital, I came to know two fine gentlemen, both of high quality education. One was a civil engineer who I mentioned earlier, and the other a mineral engineer who worked for the Ford Motor Company in a very responsible position in their steel production area. Both of these gentlemen suffered nervous breakdowns and ultimately became hospitalized in our institution. Tragically, both committed suicide. One did so while still a patient, the other after going back into society. Neither ever exhibited any signs of insanity in my recollection, only depression, which I suspect was brought about largely through association with other mentally ill people.

I saw changes in mental health treatment systems from strictly custodial care and early psychiatric analysis to electro-shock therapy and the beginning of chemotherapy, which revolutionized treatment programs. Eventually, institutional care was exchange for small units in society, and this abandonment came at a time when institutionally trained personnel in all fields of psychiatry were peaking in treatment facilities. Granted, that the programs were successful to the point of so many recoveries that the need of sizable institutions was not feasible. This change of treatment meant that many small unit structures, such as a family care home, nursing homes or private homes, lacked the skilled personnel, but did not hire these personnel in their dismissal from large facilities.

As I see it, there will always be a need for institutional housing for some of the more severely mentally ill, and those who cannot and do not respond to present-day treatment. These people are at present wandering the streets harming themselves. Sadly, too, drug addiction plays a role.

I find it very hard to put into words how I feel about my earlier years at this hospital. Often when asked what it was like, I'm sure my answer is still inadequate. What prevails above all else is the quietness of the area and the camaraderie between the employees and between employees and patients, and yes, even between patients. And, of course, the beauty of the area and my contribution to its preservation still exists.

Appendix A-Personnel

Dr. J. D. Munson - Superintendant - 1885-1924

Dr. Munson was appointed to the superintendent's position of the then Northern Michigan Asylum on November 5, 1885. He was a very gifted man who was loved totally by patients and employees alike. He did much in the development of the hospital grounds. His "beauty is therapy/work is therapy" did great things for the patients, as well as employees who worked under this concept. He established a nursing school within the hospital and established a general public hospital. He did much for Traverse City that he never received credit for. It was not widely known at that time that he owned two stores downtown, and he also owned and operated a cherry farm on the peninsula near what is now the Bowers Harbor Inn. He was married twice, and both of his wives preceded him in death. He had one son by his first wife, who graduated from Traverse City High School and upon graduation, joined the U.S. Army and perished in the Flu Epidemic of 1918. Dr. Munson retired in June 1924 and passed away in 1929 at the age of 84. I knew him personally, although I was only ten years old at the time. He always had time to talk with me when we met on the hospital grounds.

Dr. Earle Campbell - Superintendant - 1924-1926

Dr. Campbell was the superintendent at the Newberry State Hospital. Upon Dr. Munson's retirement, he took over the superintendency of the Traverse City State Hospital and was in charge from June 1924-June 1926. He was a very well-liked man, both by employees and townspeople. His family, however, was very unhappy with the move from Newberry to Traverse City and so they returned in June 1926. He had three children, two girls and one boy. The boy was one year older than me and was often a playmate of mine. After his return to Newberry, Dr. Campbell would occasionally attend superintendents' meetings in the Traverse City area and always made it a point to come into my work area to visit. This was in the 1940s and 1950s.

Dr. George Inch - Superintendant - 1926-1931

Dr. George Inch was the successor to Dr. Campbell, and his superintendency preceded my employment tenure. He was a stern task master, given to temper outbursts and not liked by employees and associates. He was promoted to the superintendency of Ypsilanti Hospital when it first opened in 1931. As usual, my father got along with all officials, especially Dr. Inch. Dr. Inch had one daughter who was in college while she was here.

Dr. R.P. Sheets - Superintendant - 1926-1956

My involvement with Dr. Sheets spanned the years of my employment between 1935-1956. I knew him in the years prior to that as a youth living with my family on the grounds. Dr. Sheets was the assistant superintendent under Dr. Inch's tenure and came to Traverse City in 1924. As disliked as Dr. Inch was, Dr. Sheets was quite the opposite, and quite well-liked during his tenure. Dr. Sheets and his family were most wonderful to our family at the time of my father's passing, and even more so to me throughout my employment. He counseled me when I was undecided in my job future. They had one daughter, Margaret Jean, with whom I still correspond regularly. An avid advocate of many of Dr. Munson's theories in mental health activities, Dr. Sheets was in charge of the institution during its greatest periods of building growth, as well as advancement in mental health programs. With Dr. Sheets retirement, Dr. Myron Nickels took the position of superintendent. Dr. Sheets suffered such a severe stroke that he was given retirement status, and passed away during his retirement years. Dr. Nickels stayed on until Dr. Sommerness took over from 1958-1972. Sadly, Dr. Nickels, accepting retirement shortly thereafter, committed suicide.

In the following years from 1958 until the institution's closure in October 1989 there were several temporary superintendents installed. Most were brought in to assist in the institutions closure.

Alfred Leland - Head Gardener - 1934-1941

Alfred Leland, assistant gardener under my father, eventually became the Head Gardener/Florist. This happened as a result of my father's passing. At that time I then moved into Mr. Leland's former position. Alfred was an Englishman, single all his life. He was an excellent gardener and florist and was a great person to work for, but not suited for a supervisory position because he just didn't feel right in giving orders to others. Consequently, he suffered a lot of impositions by others. He became seriously ill with kidney problems early on in his working days, which presented me with several opportunities to experience life "in charge," long before I was ready for such duties. Alfred had many health problems during the time he was Department Head, and these ultimately led to his suffering a fatal heart attack in May 1941. While I had learned to handle the departmental duties in his frequent absences, I filled the position for nearly a year while a replacement was sought for him. The reason I was not considered for the job was not because of inability, but due to Civil Service mandates. Management at the hospital deeply regretted their inability to hire me for this position.

Burton Fry - Head Gardener - 1942-1968

Burt was selected for the Department Head to replace Alfred Leland. He came to our department in August 1942 to check out the job. Discovering that I was the former assistant florist, he could not understand why I didn't get the job, no matter how I explained it. I often suspected that he never felt right giving me orders, though I was happy in relinquishing the supervisory position. This relief for me was short-lived. Burt, being a single man, was drafted by the military in January 1943 for World War II. Upon his return, I dropped back to my former classification. Burt was a great person to work for. With his assistance in floral culture, I was able to learn a lot, and as we entered a new era of management and the consequent beginning of closure, many changes resulted in more promotions for me. In 1968 Burt retired and the greenhouse, as such, ceased. Burt passed away in 1995.

Charles Porter - Farm Manager - 1920-1947

Charles Porter was farm manager from 1920 until his retirement in July 1947. He was in charge of all farm activities, including dairy, field crops and vegetable and fruit products, and their growth, cultivation, harvest and storage. He was quite capable, and also in charge of the greenhouses. At the inception of my father's employment, he was assigned to the farm department. The Business Executive decided at the time to relieve Mr. Porter of the greenhouse responsibilities and give them over to my father.

With my employment commencing in 1935, I became associated with him. He had two daughters who were in essence classmates in school. Mr. Porter was a stern task master with his employees. Prior to the inception of civil service to all state employees, he quite often resorted to hiring or firing as a method of employee management His entire family, except for one daughter, has passed away.

Willard Stone - Farm Manager - 1947,
Grounds Maintenance Supervisor - 1957-1972

Stone assumed Farm Supervisory duties in July 1947, when the department was slowly undergoing abandonment. This was a difficult time to be a supervisor. Because of the changes, it was hard to gain control over department employees who constantly resented his orders. To some extent these orders were not his wishes, but the fact that he wasn't a good boss didn't help. In 1957, the farm was totally abandoned, and employees were laid-off or transferred into other departments. With all the changes, I was promoted to a Groundsman A classification, as was Willard. Other former farm employees who were not laid off or transferred became the employees of the new Grounds Maintenance Department. Willard retired in October 1972. I then became department head and stayed there until I retired in March 1984. The institution was in the process of closure, but this took several years to do.

Marie Moon - Chief Dietitian - 1919-1972

Mrs. Moon was widowed and became employed in 1919 as Chief Dietitian. She was very efficient in position which became evermore apparent as the institution grew in size. My responsibility to her was in supplying food elements, primarily fresh items, like vegetables and fruits for the kitchen. She was a remarkable woman, and when she retired in 1972, she was replaced by three dietitians.

Richard Coryell - Maintenance Supervisor - 1968-1979

Richard became my direct supervisor as the institution reduced in size. I retained my grounds supervisor position and I gained an additional crew that had been under Mr. Coryell's supervision. This group still remained under his "rule." At this time, as I mentioned, I retained my grounds crew. Up to this time, my relationship with Mr. Coryell had been excellent. With the changes going on within the institution, my work with Mr. Coryell became very strained. It was very difficult to say the least. The idea of having two supervisors led to much dissension within the personnel. As I look back, I have no animosity toward Mr. Coryell in that he was under tremendous pressure from all angles. This was exacerbated by constant institutional closures. Mr. Coryell had to take early retirement due to a heart attack which became fatal shortly after his retirement

Paul Hansen - Maintenance Supervisor - 1979-1984

Paul became my supervisor with the retirement of Mr. Coryell, and had this position until my own retirement in March 1984. We had the best of job relationships. He was always considerate and helpful during problem times, but he had troubles with his own personnel, again caused by constant institutional closures and layoff. He retired shortly after I did.

Mr. Jack Crawford - 1923-1961

Mr. Crawford was the Business Executive for the hospital. He assumed this position in 1923 and was instrumental in helping me to secure my job there in December 1934. though a severe alcoholic he was remarkable in his ability to run his job and office. He retired in early 1961 and died of a heart attack later that year.

Robert Mosher - Business Executive - 1961-1983

Mr. Mosher succeeded Mr. Crawford in 1961. He was very well liked by all employees and helpful to me with my problems as the closure of the hospital drew closer. Sadly Mr. Mosher developed cancer and had to take retirement in 1982. He passed away in 1983.

Tom Cyr - Business Executive - 1983-1993

Tom Cyr succeeded Robert Mosher. He was great to work for, though he had a most difficult time when the hospital was hastening toward closure. When it finally closed in October 1989, Tom took early retirement, but agreed to remain in charge while the State Mental Health Department and State Buildings Division determined what to do. Today, Tom lives on a farm in Leelanau County.

Appendix B

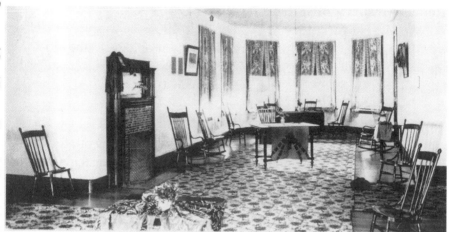

This photo was taken of cottage 24-26. This was the first of many Men's bed patient wards. It was built in 1893. The towered entry ways were removed in the early 1950s.

Photo of woman's ward. Probably early 1900's could have been hall number one.

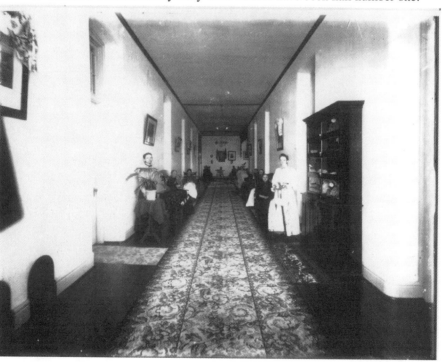

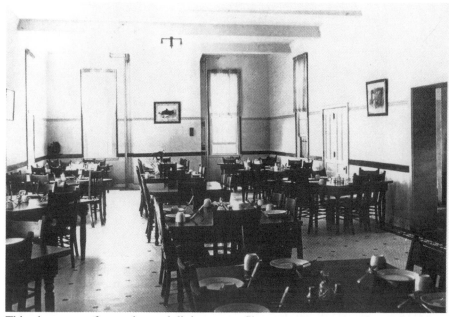

This photo was of a men's ward dining room. Six persons were seated at each table. Foreground picture gives evidence of basic table service handleless cups, metal dishware.

Photo is of barns called special barn. Housed the carriages, cutters belonging to Dr. Munson. This barn was situated near the cattle barns. Picture might have been taken in late 1890's.

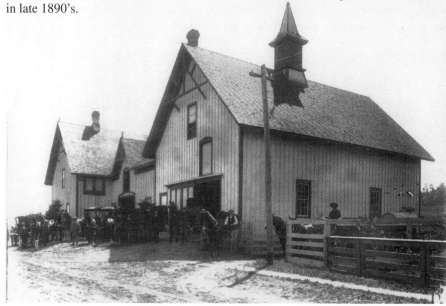

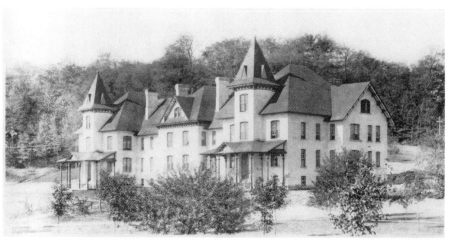

This photo was taken of cottage 24-26. This was the first of many Men's bed patient wards. It was built in 1893. The towered entry ways were removed in the early 1950s.

This is an excellent photograph of entire Building 50 as well as some of the campus. It was probably taken in the early 1900s, as prior to 1889, the campus was not in existence.

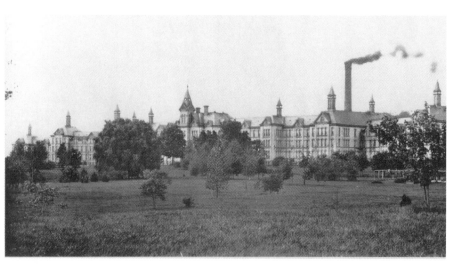

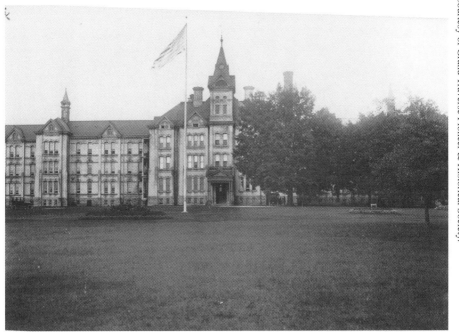

Administration and Personnel apartments of the Traverse City State Hospital.

Foreground is Cottage #28 (Men's ward) and to the left in the background is Cottage #32, also a Men's Ward, specifically a TB Unit.

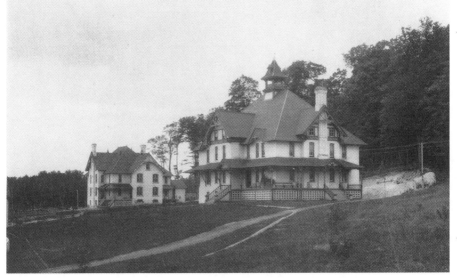

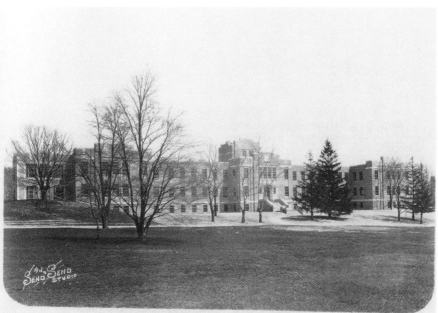

This photo, taken in early spring, is Cottage #33, which opened in 1933. This view is of the south side.

This photo shows a ward hallway decorated like a parlor. The furnishings were Victorian style.

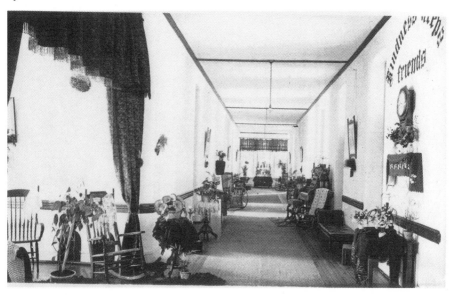

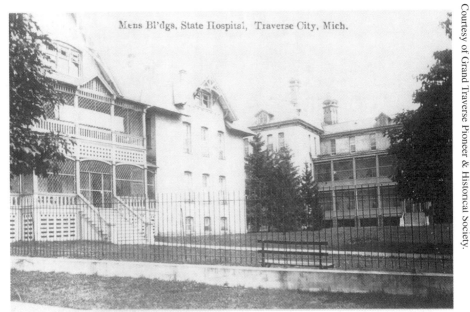

This photo taken of the west side courtyard of the Men's ward. The fenced in area allowed patients access to the courtyard. To the left is exterior of Hall 5. Directly behind this would be Halls 3, 7 and 15.

This photo, presumably taken in the early 1900s, depicts the hospital bakery and some of its employees. The trays to the left imply holiday preparation as they are filled with turkeys. These were prepared in bakery ovens.

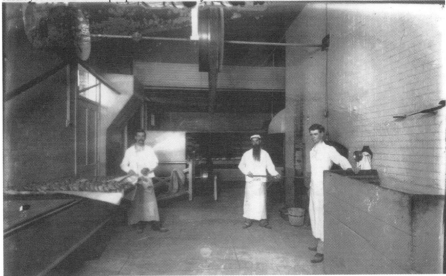

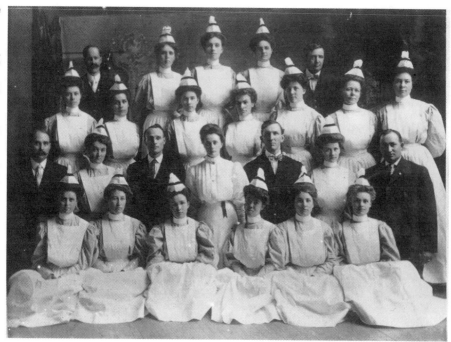

The Class of 1908, the first graduating class of nurses. Many of these graduates hired on at the hospital and I came to know them in my employment years.

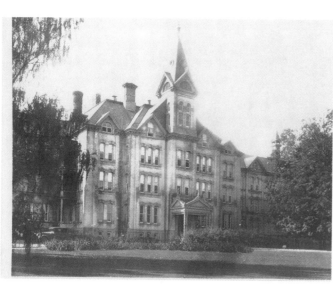

Building 50 and the Administration Building entry. The absence of bars on the windows denoted employee living quarters (on the upper floors) and the front floor was medical and business offices. The center portion was demolished in 1959 and a two story nursing office took its place.

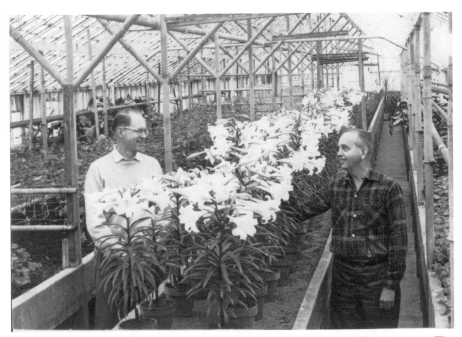

Earle Steele (left) and Burton Fry, Supervisor of Greenhouses and Garden areas. The photo, obviously within the greenhouse, was taken around 1965. The flowers, Easter lilies, were used for decor on the wards.

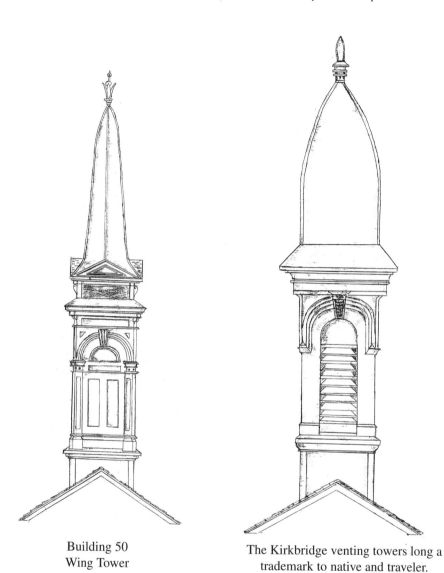

Building 50
Wing Tower

The Kirkbridge venting towers long a
trademark to native and traveler.

illustrated by Earle Steele.

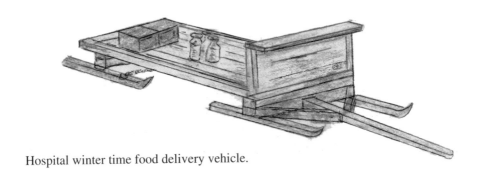

Hospital winter time food delivery vehicle.

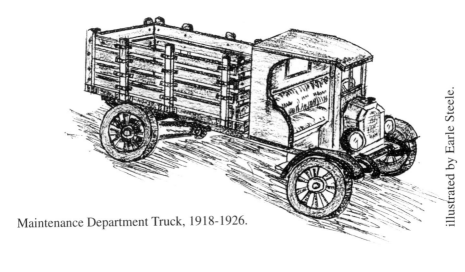

Maintenance Department Truck, 1918-1926.

illustrated by Earle Steele.

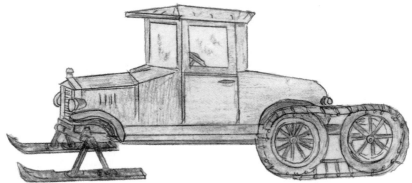

This type of vehicle was used for winter travel, primarily by physicians on country "house calls."

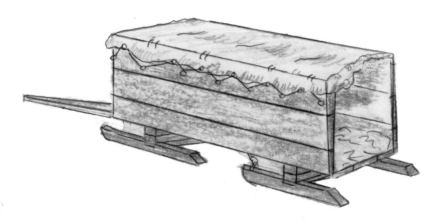

Winter-time 'school bus' for children of State Hospital employees living on grounds.

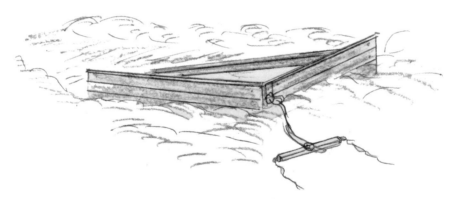

This drawing depicts a road-bed snow clearance plow constructed of a wood plank. This was generally drawn by two teams of horses driven in a tandem hitch. A similar smaller plow was utilized in the clearance of sidewalk areas. This was generally drawn by a single horse.

illustration by Earle Steele

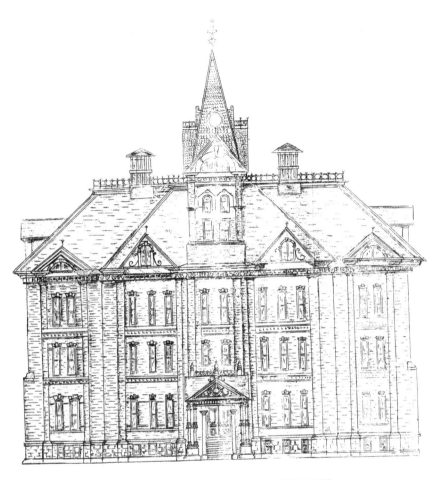

Original Administration Building 1885-1959.

illustration by Earle Steele

Earle E. Steele

Earle E. Steele was born in Farmington, Michigan on March 14, 1914. His family relocated to Traverse City when his father accepted the Head Gardner position at the Traverse City State Hospital in 1922. In 1934, he began employment with the hospital. Throughout his 49 1/2 years of employment, he served in many capacities in the greenhouse area. He spent the last 12 years of his employment as the Superintendent of the Grounds Department. He retired, with honors, in 1984. He maintained the hospital's museum from 1984 until the hospital closing in October of 1989. He has been married to his wife Marion for sixty years. They have two children, nine grandchildren and 14 great-granchildren.

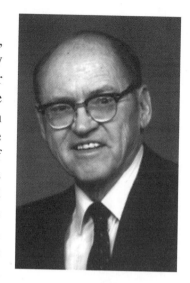

Kristen M. Hains

Kristen M. Hains is a writer who resides in Traverse City. She has always enjoyed hearing her grandfather's stories about the State Hospital and knew that someday they would write a book about it. In addition to her publishing company, Denali and Co, she is also the owner of the Stage Door Theatre Company and a co-owner of Studio 101, all located in Traverse City. Of all her titles, though, she is most proud to be "mommy" to her son Nicholas.

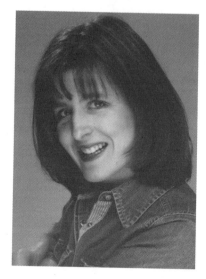